THE ANTI-INFLAMMATION DIET

How to Feel Better *and* Live Longer

JANET LEE

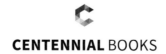

CENTENNIAL BOOKS

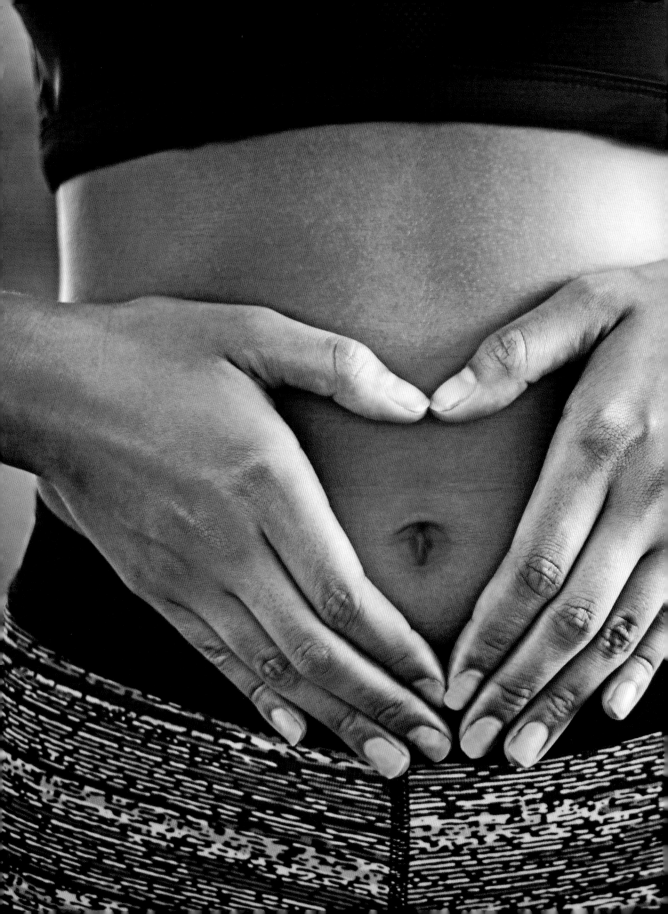

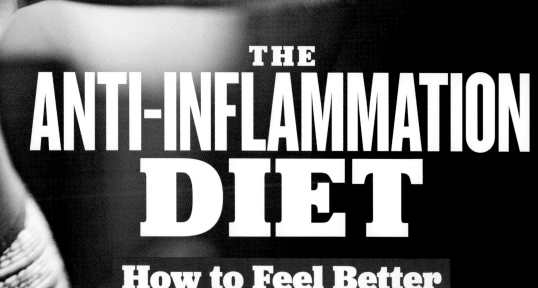

THE
ANTI-INFLAMMATION
DIET

How to Feel Better
and
Live Longer

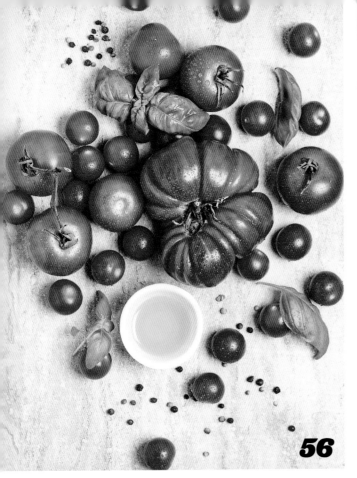

56

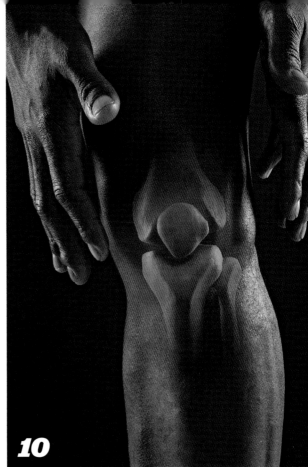

10

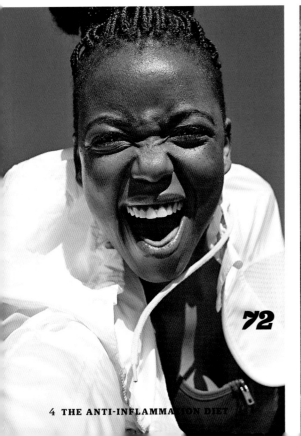

72

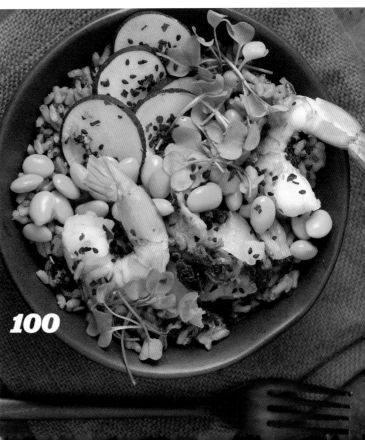

100

4 THE ANTI-INFLAMMATION DIET

Contents

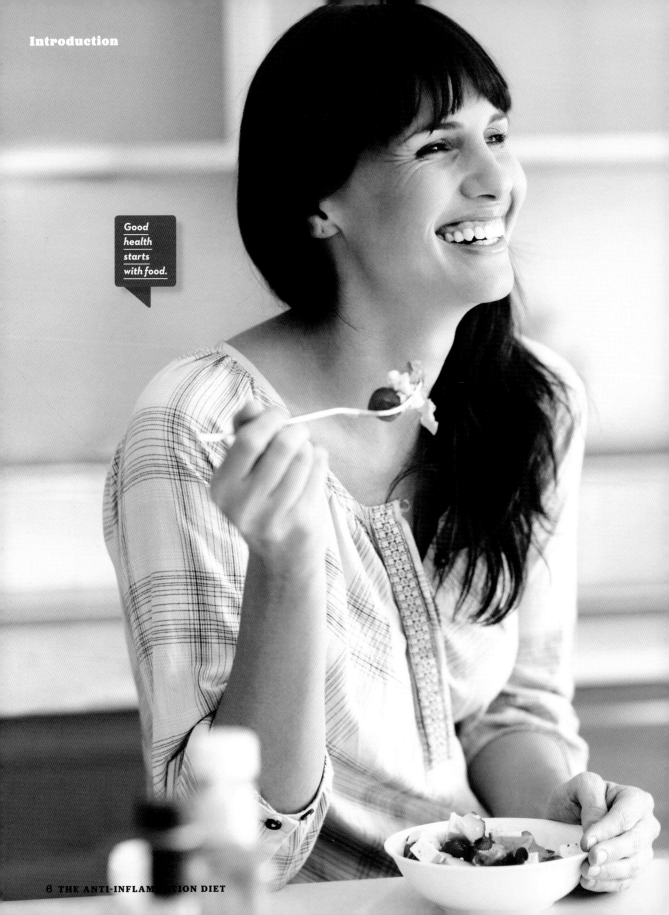

Good
health
starts
with food.

Taming the Flames

Chronic inflammation can touch every part of your body, but there's a lot you can do to quiet the uproar and boost your health.

In health care today, everyone's concerned with their stats—weight, cholesterol, blood pressure, blood sugar. You know that when these numbers are abnormal, they signal something is going wrong in the body. Lately researchers and physicians are taking a closer look at another health issue that can affect the entire body. It's preventable, but there's no specific metric associated with it. We're talking about inflammation.

Inflammation happens when the immune system flags an invader. It's one of the wonders of the human body. When anything breaches its boundaries—be it a virus, parasite or wound—the body launches its internal defense systems. Inflammation is part of the healing process. Unfortunately, things such as diet, stress and poor sleep can prompt low-level inflammation that turns chronic. It's a contributor to conditions such as heart disease, diabetes, obesity, allergies, thyroid problems, rheumatoid arthritis and even COVID-19. It can also create hard-to-decipher, annoying complaints such as skin issues, headaches, gut trouble, depression, anxiety, fatigue, brain fog and more.

In this book, you'll discover how this simmering fire gets a foothold in the body and how some very easy shifts can help douse it. You'll learn about lab testing that may help you identify markers for inflammation, surprising immune system triggers and signs of hidden inflammation that can fly under the radar.

Perhaps the biggest area of research related to inflammation surrounds the gastrointestinal tract, since 75% to 80% of the immune system resides there. The inner workings of the gut play an underappreciated role in the health of your entire body, from your brain (anxiety and dementia) to your big toe (gout). If your gut isn't healthy, inflammatory compounds can escape and cause trouble elsewhere. That's why the first step when you start encountering these problems is to clean up your diet. You'll find everything you need in this book to help you identify inflammatory foods and make healthy changes—including 53 recipes that feed your body in a way that will help you maintain internal balance.

Soon you'll be able to easily spot signs of inflammation, notice when you're not feeling your best, and be ready to take action. Those good changes to squelch inflammation will pay off with better health, less risk for chronic disease and more energy. *—Janet Lee*

Chapter 1

Fire in the Hole!

*Inflammation takes root deep inside you,
smolders and spreads, affecting
all sorts of intertwined systems.*

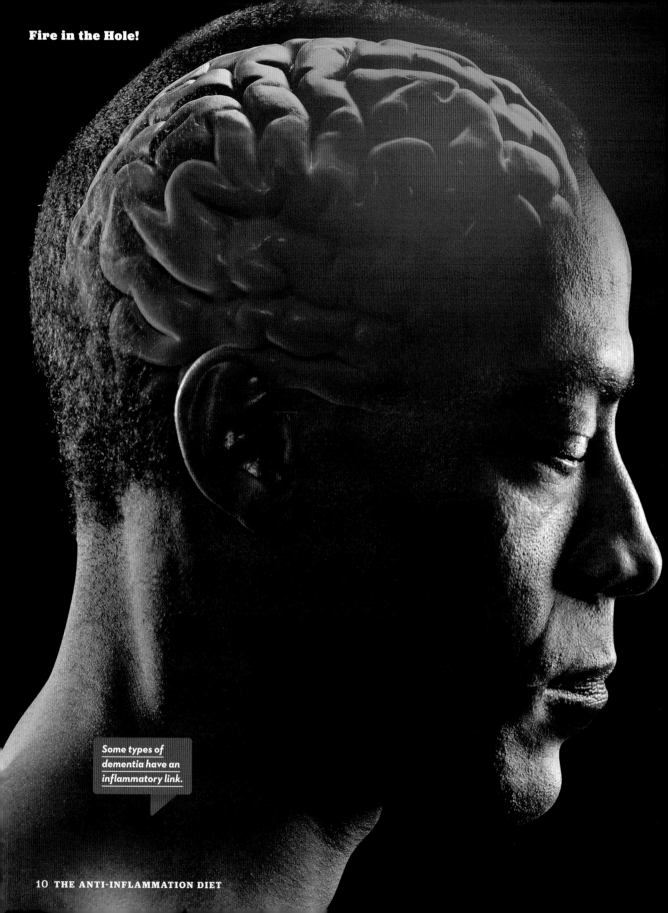

Some types of dementia have an inflammatory link.

Hot
&
Bothered

Discover what happens in your body when you have inflammation—and how it can lead to serious health problems.

R ight now, something may be going on in your body—without you having any clue—that's affecting your health. It may slowly simmer while you go about your day, unaware there's anything out of the ordinary. Eventually, though, that simmering may erupt into a full boil, and you'll start to experience health problems, large or small, that can potentially change your life.

We're talking about inflammation. Like stress,

inflammation is a natural reaction and can be beneficial or harmful. "Inflammation is a very important piece of our health. It's our body's way of telling the brain, 'Something is happening, we need help,'" says Jenelle Kim, DACM, LAc, a doctor of Chinese medicine in San Diego and founder and lead formulator for JBK Wellness Labs.

The problem arises when you ignore this missive from the body or fail to completely heal the injury, infection or other cause

of inflammation. In those instances, it can become unbalanced, flipping the switch from "good" (like in acute situations) to "bad" (chronic inflammation) and wreaking havoc on different systems of the body.

There is hope! First, by learning about inflammation and the subtle ways it reveals itself, you can get in touch with your body's signals to better know when it's affecting you. Second, by incorporating anti-inflammatory practices into your lifestyle, you can

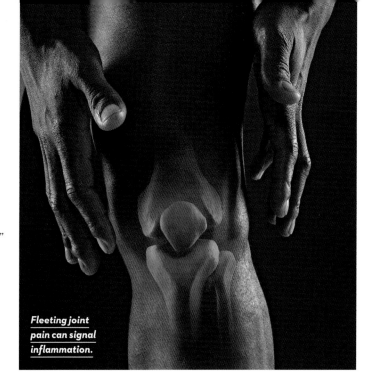

Fleeting joint pain can signal inflammation.

keep your body as healthy as possible and limit unhealthy flare-ups. "Inflammation is a really important thing to be aware of," Kim says. "If we focus on strengthening our immune system, we can balance inflammation. All it takes is little steps every day."

The 911 Call

"Inflammation is a natural response of the body's immune system," explains Aaron Hartman, MD, a functional medicine doctor in Midlothian, Virginia. "It's one of the ways in which the body responds to injuries, helping to heal them, and fights off infections." When these things happen, the immune system triggers a cascade of responses: Blood vessels dilate so more blood and immune cells can reach the affected area. In turn, that part of the body becomes red and hot to the touch (unless it's an internal infection, but even then, your temperature might go up and you may feel feverish). This process also activates pathways in the nervous system, sending messages to the brain that you're in pain, which can sometimes occur even if there's an infection. In addition, the immune cells allow more fluid into the area, leading to swelling.

"In a healthy person, these conditions flare up and then later die down and typically

WORLDWIDE, 3 IN 5 PEOPLE DIE FROM CHRONIC INFLAMMATORY DISEASES.

THE LINGO *Antigen A toxin or foreign agent that sounds the immune system's alarms.*

require no treatment, though an over-the-counter pain reliever may help relieve symptoms, a cold compress may reduce swelling, and an antibiotic may be recommended for some bacterial infections," says Jeffrey B. Blumberg, PhD, professor in the Friedman School of Nutrition Science and Policy at Tufts University

and science advisory board member for Good Pharma.

The Switch Is Stuck On

In addition to launching this standard operating procedure to activate inflammation when an injury or infection starts, the body also has a counter-mechanism to slow the inflammatory response once the triggering problem has resolved so your body can return to its normal steady state, Hartman explains. When your body can't eliminate a pathogen for whatever reason (this

When Inflammation Is a Good Thing

Although chronic inflammation can wreak havoc on the body, acute, or short-term inflammation is necessary and healthy. Besides helping to heal that sprained ankle, here are four surprising examples of times when you really want inflammation:

POST-WORKOUT
"Muscle fibers are torn during workouts, causing inflammation," explains Melanie Keller, ND. As the body repairs these tears, it causes the muscles to become stronger, in turn helping you lift more weight or do more reps of an exercise.*

FOOD POISONING
When you eat contaminated food or undercooked meat, which may contain harmful bacteria, the lining of the intestines and stomach become inflamed. "This is the body's proper response in order to signal the blood to kill the pathogen," explains Keller. This can cause symptoms of pain, nausea and diarrhea, but it's your body's way of ejecting the bug and helping your system heal.

EMBRYO IMPLANTATION
A certain level of inflammation happens when an embryo attaches to and burrows into the lining of the uterus, where it can then grow. But too much inflammation can thwart that process.

BROKEN BONES *First blood cells rush to the site. Then inflammation sets in, in two phases: The first recruits more immune cells to help, while the second phase removes debris from the area and initiates bone healing.*

can happen in the case of mononucleosis, Lyme disease and even food poisoning), your immune response "remains on for too long," Blumberg says. Your body fails to hit the brakes on inflammation and instead, the immune response continues, becoming chronic. This can also occur if you have untreated causes of acute inflammation (such as gingivitis or an injury) or are exposed long term to industrial chemicals or polluted air, says Melanie Keller, ND, a naturopathic doctor in Los Angeles.

Chronic inflammation can increase the risk of diabetes, cardiovascular disease, arthritis, Alzheimer's, bowel disease and cancers, although the exact "inflammation-disease" connection varies. For example, inflammation appears to promote the growth of plaque in the arteries (called atherosclerosis). This can lead to heart attack or stroke. Or in the case of bowel disease, researchers believe the immune system malfunctions, setting off an inflammatory response in the gut when there's nothing foreign to attack. Instead, the immune system turns on all or part of the GI tract. Additionally, "low-grade chronic inflammation, over time, can create an antibody response (the body's immune system warriors) and ultimately lead to autoimmunity," Hartman says. This is when your body makes antibodies against your own tissue and attacks it.

While not all chronic inflammation will lead to an autoimmune disease, "it can become a vicious cycle," Blumberg says.

"It may contribute to the onset of age-related diseases, and these diseases can also induce chronic inflammation." The long-term presence of immune cells such as macrophages and lymphocytes releases inflammatory proteins, growth factors and enzymes that damage more tissues in the body. This can cause the inflammation to perpetuate and spread to other areas.

Even worse, your lifestyle can cause or exacerbate chronic inflammation. Repeated exposure to environmental toxins such as pesticides and volatile organic compounds (VOCs, which are gasses that can be released into the air from things such as paint, carpeting and even toys), eating a highly processed diet and having psychological stress all contribute to inflammation.

"Stress...involves many neurochemical and hormonal alterations, activating the sympathetic nervous system and the hypothalamic-pituitary-adrenal axis," Blumberg says. "This can

> **THE LINGO**
> *Antibodies Immune cells that attack foreign invaders (or the body's own cells, in the case of autoimmune disorders).*

activate inflammatory responses throughout the body, including the brain." Because of these lifestyle stressors, our immune system has to continually respond, never getting a chance to fully repair, which causes it to break down.

How Inflammation Manifests Itself

You can usually tell when you have acute inflammation. It can cause redness, heat, pain, fever, swelling and/or loss of function in the affected area. On the other hand, many people show no outward signs or symptoms of chronic inflammation, Blumberg says. Others have subtle signs that could easily be attributed to other causes. These include:

> *Fatigue or poor sleep*
> *Muscle or joint pain*
> *Unexplained weight gain*
> *Depression*
> *Anxiety*
> *Headaches*
> *Hair loss*
> *Digestive issues such as constipation and diarrhea*

"All of these can be a different sign of a different inflammatory disorder," Hartman says. "Taken as a whole, they can seem kind of confusing, but a skillful practitioner can use these symptoms to figure out which organ systems and parts of your immune system—innate

> **THE LINGO** *Innate Immune System This is the body's top-line barrier to any foreign invaders, like a front door lock or a password on your computer. It's designed to keep obvious pathogens from gaining too much headway.*

or acquired—are causing inflammation and how to address it."

The only way to truly know if you have inflammation is a blood test, says Keller. Doctors can check your level of C-reactive protein (CRP). Our body releases more of this protein into the blood when it detects inflammation, whether acute or chronic. If your doctor rules out acute inflammation, they may send you to a specialist, such as a rheumatologist or cardiologist, for further testing to determine what's causing the inflammation, if you have other concerning signs or symptoms, Keller says. (See page 42 for more on CRP and other tests that can help get to the root of your inflammation.)

Keep the Lid On

As with most health conditions, you cannot control all of the risk factors for inflammation. Older people tend to have higher levels of inflammation, for example. This may be due to an overall greater exposure to environmental stressors over time, increased body fat (which tends to happen as we get older and also releases inflammatory molecules), or dysfunction of the mitochondria—the cells' internal engines which produce energy.

However, you can control many other risk factors, especially your diet. A large percentage of the immune system resides in the gastrointestinal (GI) tract, Hartman says. "Once you realize your immune system is the major system associated with inflammation, the gut becomes a primary place to work on it," he adds.

Both the Mediterranean and the DASH (Dietary Approaches to Stop Hypertension) diets have been shown to reduce inflammation (see page 48 for more on eating to beat inflammation). Or simply add more plants to your plate: Fruit, vegetables, nuts and whole grains contain fiber and a variety of antioxidants, which support gut health and have anti-inflammatory properties. Also, try to limit foods that promote inflammation such as

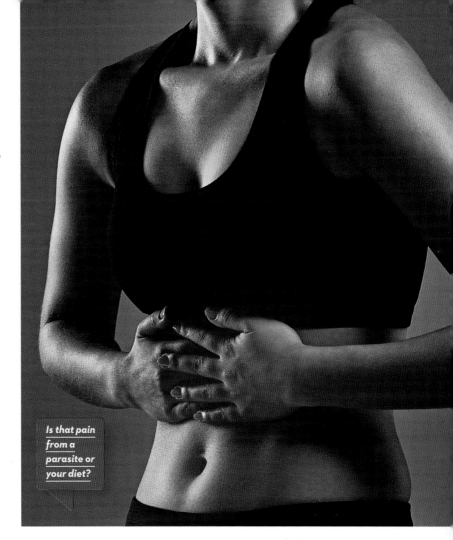

Is that pain from a parasite or your diet?

added sugars, refined carbohydrates (including white bread and pasta) and processed meats, Blumberg suggests.

Not surprisingly, regular physical activity also helps boost the immune system in a healthy way and reduces inflammation. Although it's unclear exactly why, exercise may increase levels of anti-inflammatory molecules called myokines and decrease pro-inflammatory cytokines.

Last up, you cannot neglect the importance of getting enough z's. "Poor sleep can cause inflammation, spread inflammation and prevent your body from adapting to it," Hartman says. On the other hand, consistent sufficient sleep may help lower it.

Keep reading this book for ways to spot sneaky inflammation and all sorts of lifestyle-enhancing strategies to keep it from getting a foothold in your body.

5 Signs You Have Inflammation

Your body is trying to tell you something. Are you listening?

Your body doesn't beat around the bush when it comes to short-term inflammation, such as when you cut yourself, bruise or break something or even experience allergies. It lets you know with five immediate (acute) signs of inflammation: swelling, pain, redness, heat and loss of function.

You can thank your immune system for all of it. Your body sends engorged white blood cells to the affected area, and this influx leads to redness and feelings of heat in that spot. The cells also bring more fluid, triggering swelling. As this happens, the brain receives messages that you're in pain, which translates to discomfort. All of this adds up to less function, whether that means it's harder to breathe (like if you have allergies) or you can't move a joint through its full range of motion (if you have sprained something).

Signs of chronic inflammation, though, can be subtle. It's easy to chalk them up to just everyday life (we're all fatigued, right?) or to forget that certain health conditions, such as diabetes, thyroid disorders and heart disease, have an inflammatory aspect. To help you stay as savvy as possible about the potential signs of inflammation—and how to manage them—we've put together this handy guide.

Fatigue

It's one of the most common complaints in doctors' offices, and it can be caused by many things, from the obvious poor night's sleep to more serious conditions, so needing more coffee than normal isn't necessarily a telltale sign of inflammation. But if there's no obvious reason for feeling exhausted all the time, that's a hint that something's going on.

Chronic inflammation causes fatigue because it increases the body's metabolism by up to 10%, according to a study published in *Nature Reviews Rheumatology* in December 2017. "Your body is constantly working so hard to balance the areas that it feels are in trouble," explains Jenelle Kim, DACM, LAc, a doctor of Chinese medicine in San Diego. "It has no time to rest."

At the same time, your body makes less adenosine triphosphate, or ATP, the cells' primary form of energy. Most of the time, your system uses glucose from the food you eat to create ATP. But chronic inflammation is associated with insulin resistance (cells don't want to respond to insulin) and reduced glucose tolerance, meaning the body can't produce as much ATP from glucose. So it tries to compensate by using fat and protein. These involve more complicated, longer processes to produce ATP, however, which means less cellular energy.

Lastly, back to the sleep issue. When someone has inflammation, they often don't sleep well. It can disturb your circadian rhythms (the body's "internal clock"), making it even harder to get a good night's rest and exacerbating fatigue.

Treat It The best way to deal with fatigue is to prioritize quality z's. Practice good sleep hygiene, going to bed and rising at the same time every day (even on weekends), avoiding screens (TV, phone, laptop—you name it) an hour before turning in, keeping your bedroom cool and dark, restricting activities in your bed to sleeping and sex, and avoiding caffeine in the afternoon and evening. If sleep continues to be a real struggle, consult a doctor who may recommend testing for sleep disorders.

Migraine

Many researchers believe migraine is a neuroinflammatory disease. For example, in a study of more than 400 adults published in the journal *Cephalalgia* in March 2018, scientists measured levels of high-sensitivity C-reactive

> ***ANTIANXIETY TIP***
> *If you tend toward anxiety, limit your alcohol and caffeine intake. Both can amplify feelings of panic and worry.*

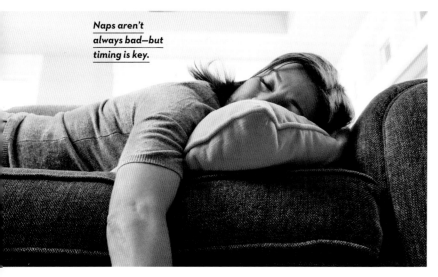

Naps aren't always bad—but timing is key.

protein (hs-CRP, a marker of inflammation) in people who experienced migraine with aura, migraine without aura and no migraine. (Migraine as a condition doesn't necessarily involve a headache; it can be aura only or manifest as vision changes or even partial paralysis.) As discovered in other studies, people who had any type of migraine also had higher levels of hs-CRP. This was particularly true in cases among young women.

It's unclear how inflammation plays a role in migraine. Some doctors believe blood vessels in and around the brain become highly inflamed, in turn triggering pain. Other researchers theorize that inflammation activates a nerve in the brain (the trigeminal ganglion nerve) that increases levels of calcitonin gene related peptide (CGRP). This triggers inflammation and causes blood vessels in the brain to dilate.

Treat It In some cases, over-the-counter (OTC) pain medications such as aspirin, ibuprofen (Advil), or combinations of caffeine, aspirin and acetaminophen (Excedrin Migraine) may help. However, prescription medication is often preferable, as these drugs may cause ulcers and bleeding in the GI tract if used for too long. To prevent

migraines, it can help to find ways to manage stress, promote relaxation, be physically active, and identify and avoid triggers, such as certain foods.

Digestive Problems

Food allergies, poor diet, stress, taking antibiotics—these can all throw off the delicate balance of the gut microbiome. "The 'bad' flora proliferates and the 'good' flora decreases," leading to inflammation, explains Diana

Girnita, MD, PhD, a board-certified rheumatologist in Palo Alto, California. This can result in symptoms including abdominal pain, unexplained weight loss, chronic diarrhea and blood or mucus in your stool.

According to a paper published in August 2019 in the journal *Microorganisms*, having more bad bacteria in the gut may increase the release of enterotoxins. This makes the intestinal wall weaker, allowing more

IN IBD, BAD GI TRACT BUGS ARE OUTNUMBERING THE GOOD.

Bowel disorders can severely impact quality of life.

harmful molecules to escape the gut and promoting inflammation inside and outside the gastrointestinal tract. This only makes things worse, as certain bacteria thrive in inflammatory environments. In turn, you become more susceptible to inflammatory bowel disease (or IBD, the umbrella term for Crohn's disease and ulcerative colitis).

Treat It Doctors typically recommend anti-inflammatories such as aminosalicylates or corticosteroids as the first line of treatment for IBD. If those don't help, immunosuppressant or biologics may help fight the inflammation and reduce symptoms.

Overall, a diet low in processed foods and sugars and high in whole foods, fiber and fermented foods (such as kefir, yogurt, tempeh and kimchi) supports a healthy gut, Girnita says. However, if you do have IBD, fiber may cause the condition to flare up, so be mindful of how your body reacts to specific foods and keep a food journal to help identify triggers.

Eczema

Also called atopic dermatitis, eczema causes dry, itchy skin. All that itching then leads to redness, cracks, sensitive skin and bumps that leak clear fluid.

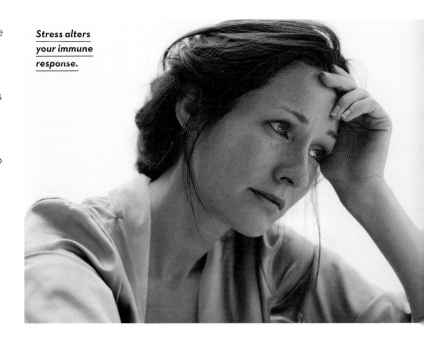

Stress alters your immune response.

NEW RESEARCH LINKS CERTAIN GUT BACTERIA WITH ANXIETY.

While experts still don't know exactly what causes eczema, genetics, environmental factors (such as low humidity, harsh soaps and air pollutants) and immune dysregulation appear to play a role. It's believed that the immune system overreacts to triggers from outside or inside the body and jump-starts the inflammatory process, resulting in changes in the skin.

Treat It Self-care may be enough to manage eczema. Moisturizer or hydrocortisone can keep skin dry and reduce the urge to scratch. Antihistamines and colloidal oatmeal baths may also help, as can avoiding detergents, soaps and fabric that irritate skin. Or try wet wrap therapy: After bathing, pat dry and apply moisturizer or medical creams. Then wet a piece of gauze and wring it out so it's damp. Place this on the affected area and cover with dry gauze. Leave the wraps on for several hours or even overnight. If none of this works, talk to your doctor about prescription options.

Anxiety

Mental health disorders are typically complex conditions with several underlying causes. That said, inflammation may play a role in anxiety in two ways. First, an estimated 90% of serotonin (the hormone that regulates mood) is made in the gut. If the gut becomes inflamed, it can decrease production of serotonin, potentially contributing to anxiety, explains Lauren Deville, NMD, a naturopathic doctor in Tucson, Arizona. Second, stress causes the hypothalamus in the brain to produce endorphins. Once endorphins reach a high enough level, we feel less stress, Deville says. But chronic inflammation doesn't allow this benefit to happen; instead, long term lower levels of endorphins and the perpetuating stress response lead to depression but also potentially anxiety, she says.

Treat It The best way to address anxiety is to work with a licensed therapist, psychologist or psychiatrist. Cognitive behavioral therapy (CBT) is the gold standard for treating anxiety. It helps you learn how to identify and challenge distorted thoughts. Medication may also help.

Squelch Possible Problems

No matter what hints—or clear alarms—your body is giving that you may have inflammation, some basic healthy practices have been shown to help reduce any inflammation. The first thing to try: Eat as clean as you can with a diet rich in a variety of whole foods. Also make sure you're getting regular physical activity and find some ways to manage your stress. Keep reading for more how-to strategies on each of these subjects!

Can You Blame It on Your Genes?

With many inflammatory conditions—including rheumatoid arthritis, atherosclerosis (the buildup of plaques in the arteries of the heart), hypothyroidism, IBD and psoriasis, to name a few—having a family member who's been diagnosed means you're at greater risk of also having that condition. But is there a genetic link for general inflammation? Unfortunately, it's not that simple.

The short answer is no. At this point, researchers have not identified any one genetic marker that makes someone more prone to inflammation. We do, however, know that certain genes control the pro- and anti-inflammatory responses that the body activates when it detects an invader. And everyone's response is different. That's in part because genes aren't the only variable that affect your health and risk of disease. Environmental and lifestyle factors such as the air quality where you live, whether you smoke, how active you are, and your diet all play a role in the development of inflammation—and these are the first things you should address when trying to eradicate inflammation.

So even if you could test and find out if you had an "inflammation gene," it wouldn't mean you're destined to develop it. But by taking action to tip the lifestyle factors you can control in your favor, you could prevent possible inflammation from happening. (The same holds true if you have a genetic predisposition to heart disease, diabetes and dementia.)

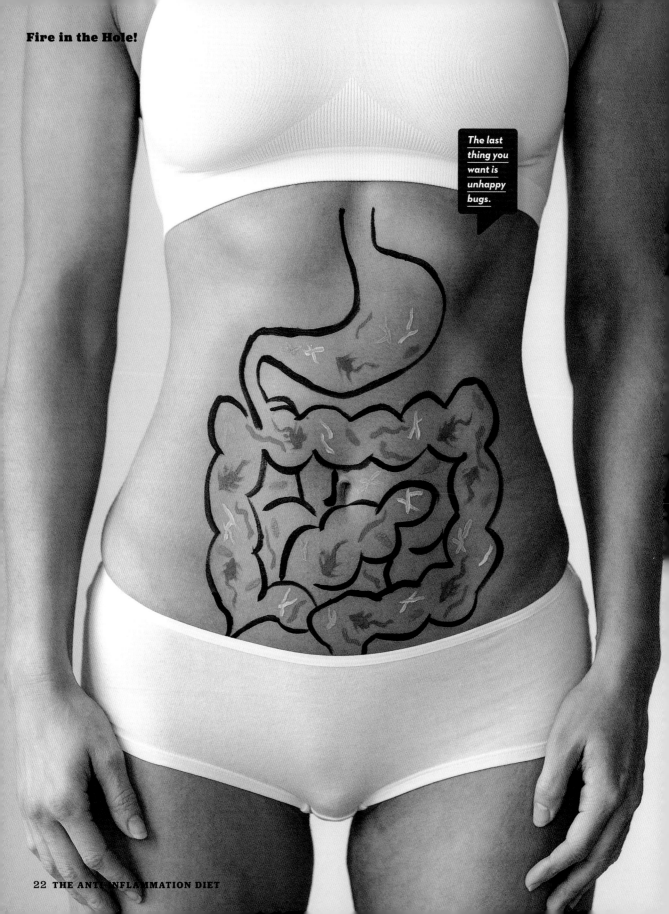

GUT Reactions

Those microscopic bugs in your GI tract have an outsize role in triggering system-wide inflammation.

Pain, gas, bloating, constipation— part of a normal day, right? Not so fast. Before you blame that tendency toward heartburn or irritable bowel on your genetics (or your love of burritos) and assume you're doomed to a life of gut trouble, take some time to understand what's really happening. These symptoms are, in fact, valuable signals from your body, alerting you that something is off-kilter.

Of course, those are the more obvious gut-related symptoms and they're the ones we write off as just part of being human. Anxiety, depression, fatigue, asthma, rashes, acne and autoimmune diseases such as Hashimoto's and rheumatoid arthritis are other signs of GI trouble. They illustrate how what happens in the 25 feet or so of the digestive tract can cause a far-reaching inflammatory response.

When Your GI Tract Springs a Leak

The small intestine is the longest section of your gastrointestinal tract: It's about 15 to 20 feet in length, depending on the person, and approximately an inch in diameter. Your body absorbs nutrients from your food, including electrolytes, minerals, vitamins and amino acids, through the intestinal epithelium—a single-cell-thick layer that forms a barrier between what's in the GI tract and the rest of the body. These cells prevent entry of potentially harmful substances into the body, including bacteria, fungi, parasites and viruses.

"Imagine your small intestine like a long tube lined with cheesecloth so only the healthy nutrients can pass through it with ease into your blood to nourish it," says Great Neck, New York-based Carla Alpert, FDN-P, a board-certified functional medicine health coach specializing in gut health and the owner of Well Humans.

Next, Alpert suggests we imagine those holes in the cloth getting bigger. Now things are sneaking through that would normally not leave the small intestine—larger particles of undigested or partially digested food, as well as microbes. This is called increased intestinal permeability (the medical term), aka "leaky gut."

The body's response? It sends white blood cells to battle the invaders, causing what's known as an inflammation cascade, where inflammation occurs both locally (in the small intestine) and systemically in other parts of the body, such as the joints and brain (see sidebar). With leaky gut, "the immune system is working overtime and is eventually dysfunctional," Alpert says.

Another way to think of leaky gut is like a door, says Lacey Dunn, RD, LD. Based in Jacksonville, Florida, Dunn is the founder of UpliftFit Nutrition and author of *The Women's Guide to Hormonal Harmony*. The door works well if it's not being compromised by food intolerances, chemicals that interfere with hormone production in the body (endocrine disrupters) and stress. If there is stress, mold toxicities, nutrition deficiencies and other problems, to name some common issues, the door becomes damaged and won't close as easily or tightly as it used to.

This immune reaction in the body can possibly even lead to autoimmune diseases. According to an article published in the journal *Frontiers in Immunology*, "multiple diseases may arise or be exacerbated due to a leaky gut...including inflammatory bowel disease, celiac disease, autoimmune hepatitis, Type 1 diabetes, multiple sclerosis and systemic lupus erythematosus."

Vicious Cycles

The vagus nerve is the 10th cranial nerve (coming from the brain and winding all the way down to the abdomen) and serves as an information highway between the brain and gut—a two-way street of communication that impacts every aspect of gut function, says Alpert. "This includes the release of enzymes, gut motility and blood flow. Constipation is a common early sign of impaired vagal nerve function," says Alpert. With constipation, the vagus nerve starts getting less information from

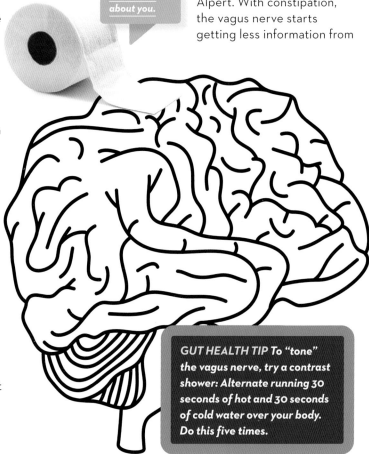

Your poop has a lot to say about you.

GUT HEALTH TIP To "tone" the vagus nerve, try a contrast shower: Alternate running 30 seconds of hot and 30 seconds of cold water over your body. Do this five times.

with serious illness. For example, "low-grade chronic inflammation caused by constipation may have an effect on the onset of fibromyalgia," according to research published in the *Annals of Rheumatic Diseases.*

ID Your Bugs

Leaky gut used to be considered a controversial "diagnosis," but it's increasingly recognized (and researched) by mainstream medicine. Some health care providers, however, including primary care providers and GI specialists, still may not acknowledge it and may offer laxatives, reflux drugs and other medicines as a way to address the symptoms instead.

When it comes to assessing gut function, Alpert says it's important to "test, never

neurotransmitters in the gut, and in turn its signals from the brain get muddled. Poor vagus nerve function triggers even more constipation.

Chronic constipation can also contribute to inflammation, because the balance of the microflora in the gut is thrown off. There might be too many bad bacteria and the bugs may be colonizing the wrong areas of the GI tract. As the bacteria break down fiber in the

EATING TOO FEW CALORIES REDUCES THE DIVERSITY OF BACTERIA IN THE INTESTINES.

food you eat, they normally create short-chain fatty acids, which protect against inflammation. By-products from bad bacteria include lipopolysaccharides, which can be pro-inflammatory. An inflamed gut is linked

guess." The tests used to gauge gut health vary, but if she had to suggest one must-do test, it would be the GI-MAP (Microbial Assay Plus) stool test. "It's a great starting place to help get an overall picture of

STRESS SUPPRESSES YOUR IMMUNE SYSTEM, ESPECIALLY ANTIBODIES IN THE GI TRACT'S DEFENSES THAT HELP FIGHT OFF PATHOGENS.

what is going on and offer information for specific healing opportunities," she says. The GI-MAP test, done via a fecal sample, can look for underlying imbalances such as bacteria or parasites, and it gives a snapshot of digestive health.

Other options, including a food sensitivity test or an elimination diet, may also be useful to figure out which foods may be causing gut reactions. Gluten, dairy, alcohol, artificial sweeteners and pain relievers such as ibuprofen are common irritants.

To get a really full picture of gut health—and how to address it—people need to be assessed for the "balance of good and bad gut bacteria, possible underlying infections like parasites or Candida (an overgrowth of a yeast that's normally present in the gut), digestion itself...nutrition and lifestyle habits, like sleep, stress reduction and movement too," says Alpert.

Healing From the Inside

One of the most common causes of leaky gut is chronic stress, says Dunn. "It suppresses your immune system and secretory IgA," she says. Secretory IgA (which stands for immunoglobulin A) is an antibody found in the intestines that serves as a first line of defense against pathogens, such as bacteria and parasites. If it's not working properly, more pathogens will get past and potentially into your system. In fact, at least 60% to 70% of our immune system resides in the gut.

Undereating and over-exercising can also cause chronic inflammation, Dunn says, because in this state, "the last thing your body wants to do is support the intestinal lining."

It's functioning more in panic mode. Undereating might also include eating a diet that's too limited. "People run the risk of nutritional deficiencies if they're eating the same, nonvaried diet every day," Dunn says.

Leaky gut is more common in women because of the fluctuations of the hormones progesterone and estrogen, Dunn says, both of which impact the gut lining. During pregnancy, for example, high levels of progesterone protect a woman's body by tightening the junctions in the mucosa of the intestinal lining, and decreasing systemic inflammation, according to a 2019 study published in the journal Nature. During menopause, both hormones drop and studies have shown microbiome diversity declines during this time.

To rebalance the gut, it's important to work on lifestyle habits, such as getting enough sleep, reducing stress and upping exercise, says Alpert. You also want to address any triggers such as infections and food intolerances, and support the microbiome with pre- and probiotics. Popping a supplement, however, without addressing underlying reasons for gut dysfunction, is not helpful. "If absorption is not working well, you can take all the supplements in the world and they won't help if your body can't assimilate them," Alpert warns.

Eating a variety of unprocessed, plant-based

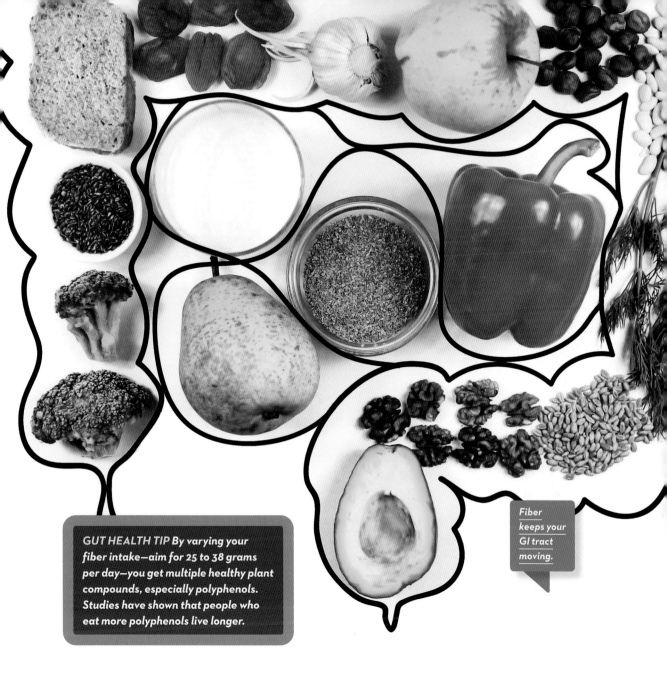

foods is also important. "A lot of people don't think about diversity when it comes to their fiber," says Dunn. But it's important because bacteria in the gut consume the non-digestible dietary fibers—present in foods such as cauliflower, spinach and blackberries—and produce important short-chain fatty acids. "The lining of the intestines degrades without the short-chain fatty acids," says Dunn, "so eat a variety of plant fiber. It's one of the best things you can do to support the gut lining and reduce inflammation."

It's clear that supporting gut health goes way beyond diet. It not only helps protect against issues such as constipation or bloating, but can help you avoid or improve inflammatory diseases.

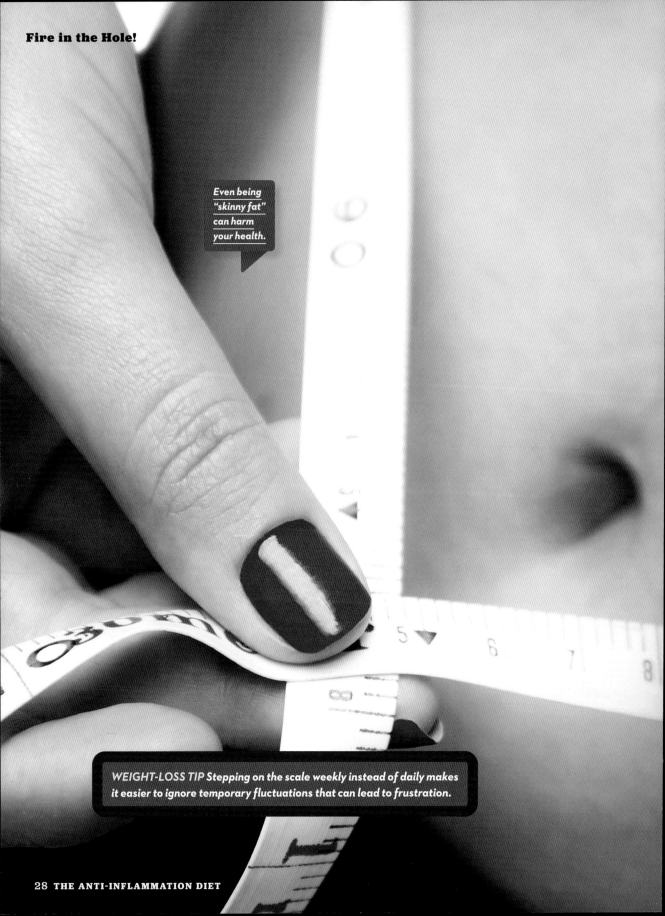

Even being "skinny fat" can harm your health.

WEIGHT-LOSS TIP Stepping on the scale weekly instead of daily makes it easier to ignore temporary fluctuations that can lead to frustration.

A Weighty Problem

The combo of extra pounds and inflammation can make it hard to battle either one.

One of the biggest causes of inflammation is excess weight—and one of the most significant causes of excess weight can be inflammation. Talk about an ugly cycle. "As body weight increases through the accumulation of fat, many systems are thrown out of balance, including the immune system," says Boston-based William Li, MD, author of *Eat to Beat Disease: The New Science of How Your Body Can Heal Itself*.

When you have excess weight, your body produces more of a certain type of fat called white adipose tissue, which doesn't just store energy, it actually plays a role in functions such as hormone regulation, hunger signals, insulin release and immune system control. This tissue causes more of a certain type of immune cell, called macrophages, to be released, which can prompt more inflammation. "Continuous inflammation stresses your organs, damages DNA and causes disruption of your gut microbiome, which itself is critical for lowering inflammation," says Li. While that's happening, inflammatory cells release growth factors that direct your fat cells to grow, which is why you're more likely to gain even more weight.

How do you break the cycle? Implementing strategies that can prompt sustainable weight loss is crucial, says Li. Rather than trying to drop pounds quickly, a better approach is to make lifestyle choices that are helpful—and healthful—in the long term.

Here are the big four:

1. Change Your Plate

Diet is the linchpin of any weight-loss program, according to all sorts of studies. Besides cutting back (sanely) on calories, look at the foods you're choosing. Eating in a way that reduces inflammation can often have the added benefit of helping you reduce body fat at the same time. That's because highly inflammatory choices—such as fried foods, sodas and desserts—tend to be high in calories and low in nutrients. According to

Boston-based dietitian Erin Kenney, RDN, choosing anti-inflammatory foods—usually also high in antioxidants—can help with insulin resistance (when your body's cells become less sensitive to the hormone,which raises blood sugar) and fat loss, and give you plenty of vitamins and minerals as well. Top picks include:

> *Fatty fish such as salmon, tuna and mackerel*
> *Green leafy vegetables such as kale, spinach, cabbage and arugula*
> *Brightly colored vegetables such as pumpkin, squash and bell peppers*
> *Whole grains*
> *Olive oil*
> *Fruits, especially berries, apples and cherries*
> *Nuts such as walnuts and almonds*
> *Spices such as turmeric, garlic and ginger*

Even coffee and tea, which contain anti-inflammatory compounds, can help protect against inflammation to some degree, says Kenney. "The benefits with foods like these go well beyond weight loss, although they may help with that," she adds. "At the same time that you're lowering inflammation and reducing body fat, you're also boosting your heart health, brain function, energy levels and more."

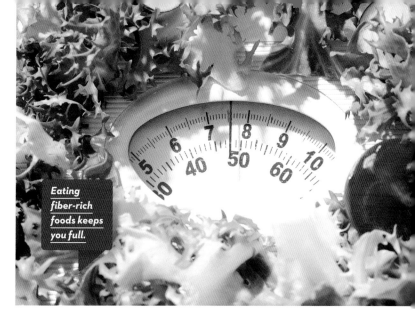

Eating fiber-rich foods keeps you full.

TO LOSE A POUND A WEEK, YOU NEED TO CUT ABOUT 500 CALORIES A DAY FROM YOUR NORMAL DIET.

2 Burn More Calories While Adding Strength

As far as physical activity goes, aerobic exercise is where the major calorie burning happens, even if it's just taking a walk every day, says Kate Ayoub, DPT, a physical therapist and health coach in Washington, D.C. If you're just getting started, find something you enjoy, and build on that. Current health guidelines recommend accumulating at least 150 minutes of exercise a week.

"Think frequency before intensity," suggests Ayoub. "Choose something you can do every day, as opposed to a hard workout that takes you days to recover from." Going on a five-minute walk after dinner and doing body-weight squats during a work break might be enough to spark a habit.

As you get more used to movement, you can add intensity, since that can play a role in weight loss too. Many studies have shown that shorter, more intense workouts (such as high-intensity interval training aka HIIT) can burn a similar amount of calories and fat as longer, moderate-paced workouts (see page 72 for more information).

Rather than focusing only on reducing fat, aim to gain lean muscle as well. Building muscle through resistance training not only helps increase strength, it can also create a permanent increase in metabolism. That makes it easier to drop pounds and keep them off.

3 Recruit a Buddy

People who join with friends and family for fitness and healthy eating tend to stay more motivated, have more fun, get some crucial social engagement and lose more weight than those who undertake an exercise program or new diet solo.

"When you're trying something new, it's so helpful to have people to support you, and who you can support as well," says Ayoub. "That might help you do a little more than you might have done otherwise, which is essential for those days you feel like giving up."

4 Sleep It Off

"Ample research backs up the importance of quality sleep for weight loss and weight management, which can have a huge impact on inflammation," says David Hanscom, MD, a former orthopedic surgeon in Seattle who now focuses on pain management methods like meditation, exercise and stress relief. Lack of sleep also alters hunger hormones.

The Dangers of Visceral Fat

When it comes to losing weight, it's really about changing your body composition: dropping fat and increasing muscle mass. But not all fat is the same—there's one type, called visceral fat, that's shown to be much more problematic than what's known as subcutaneous fat, the kind that's just under your skin.

Visceral fat accumulates deeper in the body, wrapped around, and sometimes even infiltrating, your organs. As a result, it's considered the most dangerous when it comes to your health. A study in the journal Obesity found that people who had the most visceral fat were more likely to die earlier than those who had less of the dangerous flab. That's because it can significantly raise inflammation, which has been associated with chronic conditions such as heart disease, Type 2 diabetes and more.

It's tough to know how much of this fat you have without imaging that can look at the various tissues in your body, but if you tend to carry fat in your belly, that's a warning sign. A quick waistline measurement can also sound the alarm. Anything over 35 inches for women and 40 for men is unhealthy. Fortunately, the same strategies you'd use to lower inflammation through weight loss also work for reducing visceral fat.

Similarly, sleep can reduce stress, another big factor in the weight-inflammation cycle. Numerous studies have connected higher stress levels to increased weight gain (see page 90 for more on stress and inflammation).

Once you feel stuck in the cycle of inflammation and added weight, it can feel tough to get out, says Hanscom, and that's especially true if you feel stressed about how much weight you've gained. He prefers this mental approach instead: "Think about these new behaviors as part of embracing your health and enjoying your life, not just reducing your weight. It gives you a better perspective on why you're doing them."

The Heart of the Matter

Inflammation and cardiovascular disease are closely related—and have similar fixes.

Inflammation can cause problems throughout your entire body, and unfortunately your cardiovascular system isn't an exception.

Certain conditions such as diabetes, high blood pressure and high cholesterol can create an inflammatory response and that, in turn, can affect the heart by causing plaque buildup in the coronary arteries, says Hunter Kirkland, MD, a cardiothoracic surgeon at Cardiothoracic and Vascular Surgeons in Austin, Texas. As that plaque increases, it decreases blood flow to the heart muscle, putting you at higher risk for a cardiovascular event such as a heart attack or stroke. "These conditions put stress on the arterial walls, which leads to the inflammation," he says. "Then, as the inflammation increases, the issue can get worse."

Even if you don't have those chronic conditions, inflammation may be elevated from other causes, and it would have the same effect of narrowing your coronary arteries, says Boston-based William Li, MD, president and medical director of the Angiogenesis Foundation and author of *Eat to Beat Disease: The New Science of How Your Body Can Heal Itself*.

As if that wasn't bad enough, "the inflammatory cells that gather around plaques release enzymes and cytokines that cause further damage to the lining, creating more inflammation and damage," Li says.

Potential Triggers

Although conditions like diabetes can worsen inflammation, there are also genetic and lifestyle factors to consider, says Kirkland.

"Genetics may determine how much cholesterol you

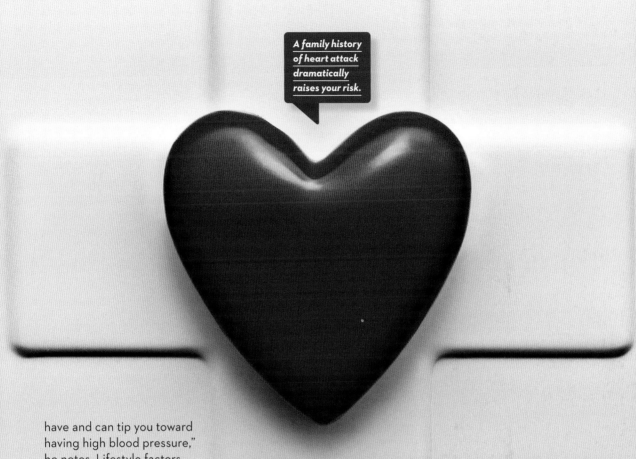

A family history of heart attack dramatically raises your risk.

have and can tip you toward having high blood pressure," he notes. Lifestyle factors such as smoking, sedentary behavior and poor diet also set you up for problems with heart disease and inflammation, Kirkland adds. (To learn more about some surprising factors that may be contributing to inflammation, see "6 Sneaky Things Fanning the Flames," page 36.)

Unfortunately, these unhealthy habits can start to add up. People who smoke are more likely to have a poor diet and are also more likely to be sedentary. That can be especially tough on the heart. And if you're

HEART-HEALTHY TIP *If you have sleep apnea, see your doctor STAT. It can significantly raise your risk of atherosclerosis.*

genetically prone toward high blood pressure, but also smoke, don't exercise, and have childhood trauma and chronic stress, all of that can keep your inflammation elevated too, says David Hanscom, MD, a former orthopedic surgeon in Seattle who now focuses on pain management

through methods such as meditation and exercise.

"You can lower inflammation to some degree with diet and exercise, but it also helps to understand how all these other issues may be affecting you," he says. "You can eat an anti-inflammatory diet, but if you're always angry and stressed, the inflammation will still win."

It might be impossible to know every factor for inflammation and heart risk that's affecting you personally, but taking the time to consider both the physical and mental perspectives is valuable.

"Your heart health is affected by emotional difficulties, and those can drive up inflammation throughout your body," says Hanscom. "You have to realize that just putting a couple lifestyle habits into place may not be enough. It's a good start, but you need to keep uncovering

JUST 60 MINUTES OF EXERCISE A WEEK CAN IMPROVE YOUR CHOLESTEROL LEVELS.

these potential inflammation triggers to help keep your heart healthy."

Tune Up Your Ticker
Cutting back on sodium and saturated fat and getting consistent exercise are essential, but as Hanscom says, that's just a starting point. Here are some other tactics that can help:

• *Lower Stress Levels With Quick Tension Tamers* Watch a funny video, water your houseplants, play with your pet. All of these have an immediate effect on lowering stress, says Hanscom.

• *Acknowledge and Address Emotional Trauma* That may mean seeking out therapy or other types of support.

• *See Your Doc* Both blood pressure and cholesterol can be elevated without any symptoms, says Kirkland. In addition, a high-sensitivity C-reactive protein test (hs-CRP) can indicate if there's inflammation present (see page 42 for more caveats on this kind of testing). Controlling heart disease risk can lower inflammation, so your doctor

may advise you to take statins or blood pressure meds and he or she can assess your overall cardiovascular disease risk factors.

• *Get Good Z's* Insomnia has been linked to high blood pressure, heart disease and hormonal shifts that can negatively impact your weight. In addition, good sleep has a positive ripple effect on other heart health factors.

• *Up the Anti-Inflammatories* Food, that is. "In general, eating more plant-based options with high fiber, nuts, whole grains and legumes are protective for heart health," Li says. "They can even reverse coronary plaques."

It's hard to know how much inflammation is affecting your heart, says Bindiya Gandhi, MD, an Atlanta-based functional medicine physician. Most doctors won't test for inflammatory markers since they don't pinpoint the source of the problem. With the changes here, you're covering all your bases and setting up your ticker for many more good years to come.

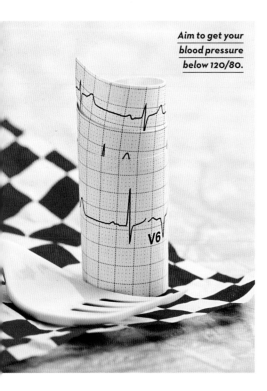

Aim to get your blood pressure below 120/80.

Anatomy of a Clot

The plaques in your blood vessels are essentially streaks of fat that accumulate on the damaged lining, says William Li, MD. That damage can happen as part of aging or from certain lifestyle choices such as smoking, poor diet and being sedentary.

As the fat layer grows, it attracts inflammatory cells that embed themselves into the fat and release cytokines—a type of protein that regulates immune function and inflammation. Think of them as a signal flare from a damaged ship, calling for rescue.

That alert brings even more inflammatory cells rushing in, along with enzymes that further damage the blood vessel lining, Li says. The growing plaque becomes a mound of fat laced with inflammatory cells, which becomes a clot.

"As the plaque expands inside the blood vessel, it narrows the space where blood flows and this causes a condition called ischemia," Li explains. "Healthy cells beyond the blockage suffer because they do not get enough oxygen, and this causes damage to the tissue. In the case of the heart, this results in chest pain or angina. In the brain, poor blood flow can impair memory and cognition."

The real problem is when inflammation within the plaque causes it to rupture. Inflammatory cells release enzymes that can cause fractures in the fatty mound. A ruptured plaque can break off pieces of the clot that can flow downstream in the blood vessel and cause a blockage in an organ. When this occurs in the brain, it causes a stroke. When this occurs in the heart, it can cause a heart attack.

"If a plaque ruptures in a particular way such that one side of the plaque is swinging free and the other side is still tethered to the main plaque, the free part can act like a trapdoor and completely seal off the blood vessel, cutting off blood flow," Li adds. "This can lead to a severe heart attack."

As this is happening, the presence of the plaque will continue to attract more inflammatory cells, leading to further damage.

To reverse this progression, your doctor will likely recommend lifestyle changes and possibly even medication. If the damage is severe, you could be a candidate for a surgical intervention like a stent or possibly even a bypass if the artery is significantly blocked. Even with a newly opened artery, eating better, quitting smoking, reducing sodium and other lifestyle shifts will help reduce inflammation and ensure that your other arteries don't have the same problem.

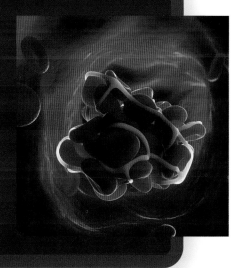

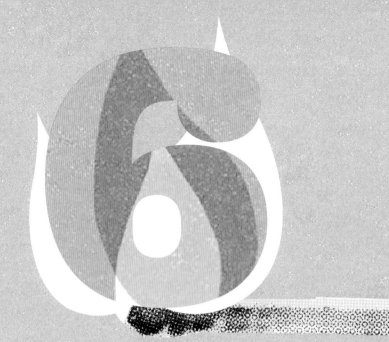

6 Sneaky Things Fanning *the* Flames

You might be setting the stage for health issues with these "matches."

Allergies are a type of *chronic inflammation*.

I nflammation can trigger numerous health issues, from autoimmune diseases to cardiovascular problems. There are obviously some major contributing factors behind the inflammatory response—poor diet and sleep and uncontrolled stress being three biggies—but there are some lesser-known culprits at play as well. These sneaky saboteurs might normally fly under your radar, but now you'll know what to look for—and snuff out fast.

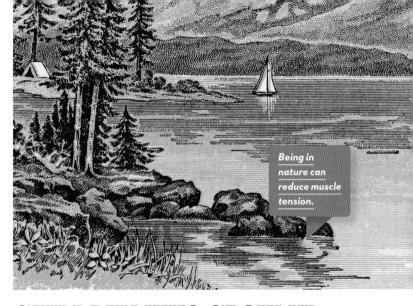

Being in nature can reduce muscle tension.

1 Childhood Trauma

Could what happened to you as a kid really affect your health decades later, even if you've moved on? Absolutely, says David Hanscom, MD, a former orthopedic surgeon in Seattle who now focuses on pain management through non-surgical methods such as meditation, exercise and stress relief.

"The way we learned to react to situations as children is a big deal when it comes to inflammation, because the inflammatory process is easily triggered by stress," he says. "If you've been conditioned to be on high alert at all times, your body will respond by always being ready to deal with a sustained threat."

This can happen with any type of trauma, he adds. If you got in a bad car accident and now flinch whenever you come to a stop sign, that will create a surge of stress and, subsequently, an inflammatory response in the body. Childhood trauma is different, though, Hanscom

CHILDREN WHO GROW UP UNDER EXTREME STRESS HAVE MORE CHRONIC HEALTH PROBLEMS.

says, because that sudden spike doesn't recede. You're always in a "seeking safety" mode even if you're not aware of it.

"For some people, it can be enough to counteract inflammation through diet, exercise and quality sleep, but for those who've experienced trauma, these are only short-term fixes," he notes. "You need to get at the root of your inflammation, and that means seeking some help to process through your trauma and relearn how to deal with stressors. The good news is that this type of therapeutic work can have a major effect, not just on inflammation but also on overall emotional health."

2 Your Neighborhood

Similar to childhood trauma, your stomping ground can lay the seeds for inflammation if you feel threatened there. If you're in a place where there's very little green space, there's unrest or crime, or you simply feel unsafe, that can keep you in a state of heightened alarm, Hanscom says. Pollution and environmental toxins can trigger inflammation as well—which means sometimes you might have several issues layering on top of one another.

"Obviously, it's not easy to say that if you feel unsafe, you should just move, because not everyone has

HEALING TIP
A technique called Eye Movement Desensitization and Reprocessing (EMDR) may help heal trauma.

that ability," he says. "But you can become more aware of how your environment is affecting you."

Counteract the negative with regular visits to parks or by taking nature walks outside your neighborhood, joining an organization that's working toward positive shifts in your area, and even just meeting your neighbors and discussing your concerns.

Often, Hanscom adds, people can reduce the feeling of being unsafe by taking control and working toward meaningful change. Not only can that help to

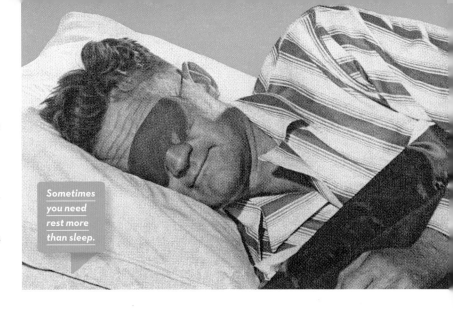

Sometimes you need rest more than sleep.

> **HEALTHY-HOME TIP**
> *To reduce pollution in your house, keep floors clean and limit fragrances such as those from candles or air fresheners.*

make a neighborhood better for everyone, but it can help your physical and mental well-being along the way.

3 Your To-Do List

Just like stress can drive up inflammation, so can lack of rest. According to a study in *Arthritis Research & Therapy*, it becomes an ugly cycle because the resulting fatigue can then worsen inflammation and any subsequent symptoms such as pain and depression.

And we're not just talking about getting a good night's sleep. Rest and sleep are not the same thing, according to Menlo Park, California-based Alex Soojung-Kim Pang, PhD, author of *Rest: Why You Get More Done When You Work Less*. Truly restorative moments aren't the kind you take only when you feel exhausted—they actually help prevent that type of depletion. Think of it as filling up your gas tank before you're only a few miles from running out of fuel.

"Many people think of rest as something they should do when they're about to collapse," says Pang. "But if you build in rest breaks to your schedule in advance, you can avoid getting to that point."

Meaningful rest is better achieved through gentle movement, deep breathing, limiting distractions and being more mindful. A short walk between work tasks can feel like a reset. So can eliminating multitasking and focusing solely on one thing at a time. In fact, integrating several restful moments into each day trains your brain to expect them, adds Hanscom. That provides some remodeling in your nervous system to tamp down your stress response.

4 Food Allergies

The most triggering dietary choices for inflammation are fatty fried foods and sugars, says Bindiya Gandhi, MD, an Atlanta-based functional medicine physician, but so-called "bad foods" aren't the only potential ones to watch.

"If you're allergic or intolerant to certain foods, that can create inflammation,"

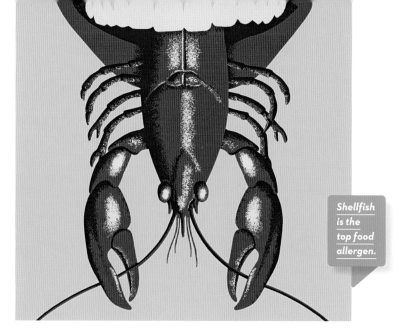

she says. "Sometimes, it's not so obvious because you may just be sensitive to some foods but not enough to have an allergic reaction."

The most likely culprits for sensitivity are gluten, dairy, soy, shellfish, nuts, corn and eggs, she says. You might feel physical or mental changes up to a few days after eating these things. But when irritation from food sensitivity becomes chronic, the symptoms can become more severe, such as digestive issues, weight gain and painful joints. That's a sign you may be heading toward a full-blown food allergy, says Gandhi.

One strategy that can help is an elimination and reintroduction test, suggests Gandhi. For example, take all the likely culprits off your menu for at least two weeks, and then bring them back into your diet one by one. That may help you pinpoint which foods are causing deeper issues throughout your body. (A registered dietitian can walk you through the process.)

> *DIET TIP Have gas and bloating? A low FODMAPs diet temporarily limits certain hard-to-digest carbs.*

FOOD SENSITIVITIES CAN CAUSE HEADACHES, SKIN IRRITATION, FATIGUE, PAIN AND MORE.

5 Frequent Infections

Catching every cold that comes your way or still battling COVID-19 symptoms even though your body supposedly "cleared" that virus months ago is an indication that your immune system is operating under stress, says Gandhi.

Each new illness leads to the release of cytokines—substances secreted by the immune system to regulate inflammation and immunity—but they're supposed to be a short-term solution. When one viral infection after another keeps overlapping, those cytokines just keep on coming, says Gandhi. That turns into chronic inflammation. Keep in mind that these can be any type of virus or infection that triggers an immune response, including skin, eye, gum, respiratory and cardiovascular infections, she says.

If this sounds like a familiar cycle, talk with your doctor about how to improve your body's defenses, which will probably include healthy lifestyle changes, including getting plenty of rest, exercising regularly, eating a nutritious diet and reducing stress—basically, all the strategies that also lower inflammation.

6 Your Iron Supplement

This mineral has a large role in the human body, but that doesn't mean more is better. Too much, either via a supplement or poor absorption in the gut due to a GI tract disorder, can amplify inflammation in the intestines—and beyond.

People with hemochromatosis, a common genetic condition where the body absorbs too much iron, can actually overdose on the mineral. (Symptoms include fatigue—which, incidentally, can also be a sign of anemia or *too little* iron—joint pain and heart palpitations.) Always check with your doctor and get blood work done *before* you start taking a supplement that contains high doses of iron.

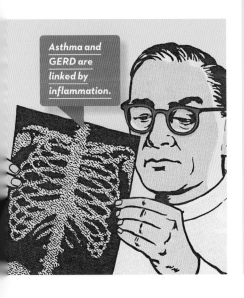

Asthma and GERD are linked by inflammation.

The Small Gland With a Big Role

Although it can affect your entire body in many ways, there are some circumstances where inflammation shows up very clearly in one system or organ. One such example is the thyroid, the bow-tie-shaped gland that sits at the lower front of your neck. "Thyroiditis" means inflammation of the thyroid gland and it's usually caused by an autoimmune condition called Hashimoto's thyroiditis. In Hashimoto's, your immune system attacks the cells of the thyroid, leading to inflammation and a lack of crucial thyroid hormones, which affect virtually every organ in the body and help regulate your metabolism.

Signs and symptoms of Hashimoto's include fatigue, puffiness in the face, feeling cold, hair loss, weight gain, muscle and joint aches and pain, depression, memory problems and menstrual irregularities. While a standard blood test can tell you if your levels of thyroid hormone are dysregulated (in the case of hypothyroidism, your TSH—thyroid stimulating hormone—levels will be elevated while some of your thyroid hormones will be low or normal), they won't tell you if you have Hashimoto's. (In some cases your thyroid levels may rise before they drop.)

If your doctor is noticing signs or symptoms of hypothyroidism and your TSH levels are on the high end of normal or higher, they may order a full thyroid panel and an antibody test to see if anti-thyroid antibodies are detectable. Even a TSH that's creeping toward the high end of "normal" may be a signal that there's inflammation because your immune system and pituitary are working overtime to try and get you back in balance, says Benjamin O'Donnell, MD, an endocrinologist at The Ohio State University Wexner Medical Center.

Medication and dietary changes can help get your thyroid back into the normal range and reduce inflammation.

Testing, 1-2-3

A little investigation can help reveal some potential evidence of inflammation.

*TESTING TIP **Always ask before your appointment if you need to fast (no food or drink for eight or more hours) for your blood work.***

When you're worried about your heart health, you get blood work to check your cholesterol levels. When you're worried about diabetes, you check your glucose and HbA1c. But when you have inflammation—or are worried you have it—the standard blood work isn't as helpful because it tells you nothing about the source of the inflammation, in general. That's where it takes some sleuthing and some more detailed testing, says Marzena Slater, MD, a practitioner at Root Functional Medicine in Grand Rapids, Michigan.

"I like to tell my patients that inflammation isn't just this on/off switch. It's more like a dimmer switch. There are lifelong contributors that push the switch to the inflammatory process," she explains. "We listen to their whole history to identify possible contributors to inflammation throughout their life."

As far as figuring out if there's inflammation and where it's coming from (or what it's potentially hurting, such as your arteries or gut), there are some standard blood tests as well as some specialized functional medicine tests (see sidebar, page 45) that can help narrow the source. (Note: Your doctor will discuss normal levels for each of these tests based on your health. Also note that not all of these tests are covered by insurance, so check with your doctor first.) You can easily go down the testing rabbit hole, especially if your signs and symptoms are complex, but these are a good starting point.

Insulin (Fasting) This hormone is responsible for shuttling sugar out of the blood and into the liver and muscles, where it can be stored for easily accessible fuel. When insulin starts to rise too high, that's a sign that the cells are becoming resistant to the hormone.

The pancreas tries to release more to overcome the resistance. (Eventually the beta cells in the pancreas get tired of working so hard and start slacking off.)

Inflammation can contribute to insulin resistance, especially when there's excess weight involved (such as obesity). Likewise, insulin resistance can also cause inflammation. "Insulin resistance is underdiagnosed," says Slater. "When it's caught early there's a lot we can do about it. Fasting insulin goes up sooner than fasting blood sugar goes up, so it's the first sign. It shows that the pancreas is working harder. Your insulin comes

The blood is a window to inflammation.

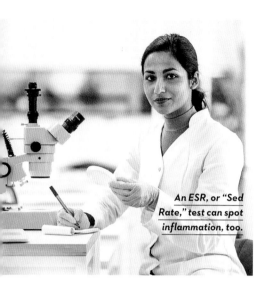

An ESR, or "Sed Rate," test can spot inflammation, too.

THE HbA1c TEST TRACKS AVERAGE BLOOD SUGARS OVER THREE MONTHS.

around, knocks on the cell door and says, 'let glucose in.' If more is around, cells don't want anymore. Insulin comes and starts knocking louder and louder."

Glucose When you eat or drink something with carbohydrates, which are just chains of sugar molecules, sugar enters your bloodstream during the digestion process. When blood levels of glucose remain high, the blood gets "sticky" and it affects everything in the body, from brain function to nerve sensitivity in the fingers and toes.

While fasting blood sugar levels below 99 are considered "normal," some doctors believe anything in the 90s is a signal that there's insulin resistance happening. Slater says 70 to 85 is optimal. "If it's higher

than that, we'll look at fasting insulin."

Oxidized LDL Cholesterol "This is a specialized test that can be a marker for inflammation," says Slater. When it's high, this can signal there's a buildup of cholesterol in the arteries. In addition, the ratio of triglycerides to HDL (good cholesterol) can signal insulin resistance.

hs-CRP C-reactive protein is a marker in the blood that increases when there's inflammation in the body, "but it doesn't tell us where the inflammation is coming from," says Slater. "The high-sensitivity (hs) test can be used to assess cardiovascular risk in people."

A 2019 research review in the journal *Molecules* noted: "Numerous studies have also reported that elevated CRP levels correlate significantly with the incidence of cardiovascular complications in patients without any symptoms of overt cardiovascular disease, as well as in patients with unstable angina, myocardial infarction, ischemic stroke, or peripheral artery disease."

WBC (White Blood Cell) A CBC, or complete blood count, tells you the amount of lymphocytes, monocytes and neutrophils (aka white blood cells) in the blood (along with other cells). WBCs are charged with attacking foreign pathogens, such as viruses. Chronically elevated WBCs have been linked with Type 2 diabetes and coronary artery disease—two inflammatory conditions—among other chronic disorders. White blood cells are what's called an acute phase reactant, says Slater, meaning they go up significantly when there's inflammation.

Omega-3 Index This measure tells you the ratio of anti-inflammatory omega-3

TESTING TIP There are more specialized tests that can potentially flag inflammation, but many haven't been validated yet.

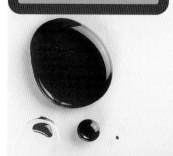

fatty acids (found in some cold-water fish, walnuts and flaxseeds) to omega-6 fatty acids (found in vegetable oil, red meat, dairy and seafood). While omega-6 acids can be beneficial in the body, we tend to get too many in our diet, which can make them pro-inflammatory. "Especially if you have allergies, chronic pain or autoimmune issues, you want to limit the amount of 6s in your diet," Slater says. Aim for a 4:1 ratio of 6s to 3s in your diet, she suggests.

Ferritin This is the storage form of iron, so it can tell you what your levels are of this crucial mineral, but that's not all. "Ferritin is another acute phase reactant, meaning it's a marker that rises when there's inflammation," says Slater.

Stool Microbiome Test You (or your doc) send your poop to a lab to look for something called fecal calprotectin, an inflammation marker in the colon, says Slater. "It can be helpful for differentiating between inflammatory bowel disease and irritable bowel syndrome," she says.

Eosinophil Protein X Eosinophils are white blood cells. This protein is a marker of eosinophil-driven inflammation, which might happen in the gastrointestinal tract if there's an allergic reaction, like to food, says Slater.

Secretory IgA (SIgA) Another stool-based test, "low SIgA can be a sign of a suppressed immune system in the GI tract and leaky gut," say Slater. "IgA (immunoglobulin A, a type of immune cell) is the first line of defense against toxins and overgrowth of bacteria and helps support the lining of the gut. If it's too high, it can be a sign of an upregulated immune system that may be fighting off dysbiosis or infection."

Should You Try Functional Medicine?

Functional medicine practitioners—who can be MDs as well as nutritionists, chiropractors, acupuncturists and naturopathic doctors—go beyond traditional blood work and levels to try to uncover the cause of disease and even spot it before it gets worse. While a standard thyroid lab test may allow for a range of 0.5 to 4 for TSH (thyroid stimulating hormone), a functional screen might cap that number at 2.5 or 3. The same goes for blood glucose. Most labs flag a level of 100 or higher as prediabetes, but eyeing those numbers before they hit that mark can tip you off that insulin resistance is happening. The goal is to catch a problem before it gets a foothold.

A two-year study performed at the Cleveland Clinic compared health-related quality of life scores in patients who were seen in the Center for Functional Medicine to those seen by normal primary care doctors. After six months, a third of patients in the functional medicine group reported increases in their quality of life and physical health of 5 points or more, compared to 22% of primary care patients. (All functional medicine patients are required to see a registered dietitian and health coach and may also meet with a behavioral health therapist.)

While more health providers are including functional medicine in their practice, it may not be covered by insurance, so check with your doctor about fees.

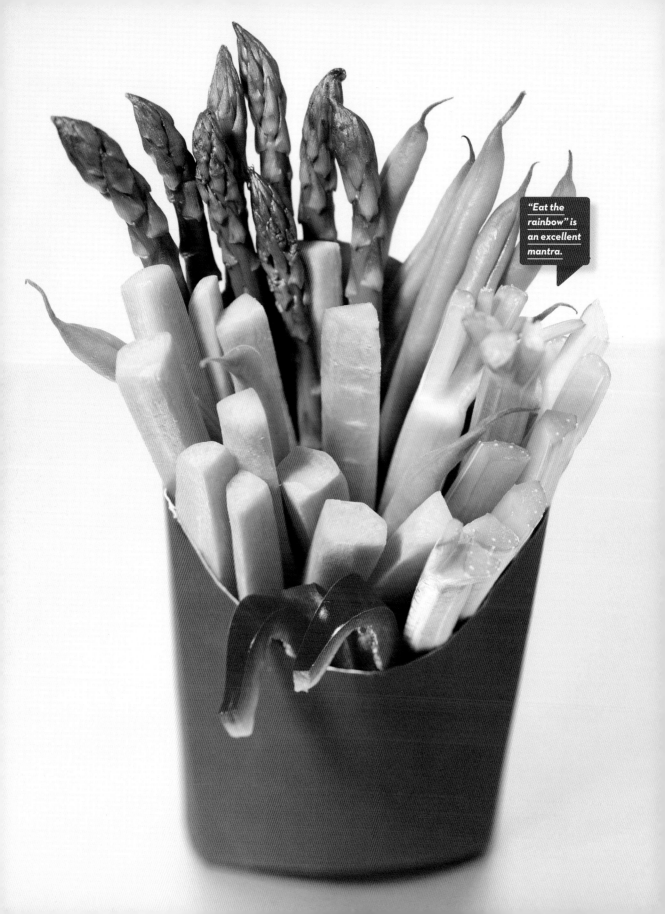

"Eat the rainbow" is an excellent mantra.

Chapter
2

The Healthy Plate

The best way to fight inflammation is with nutrient-rich whole foods that create the building blocks for systems that work well.

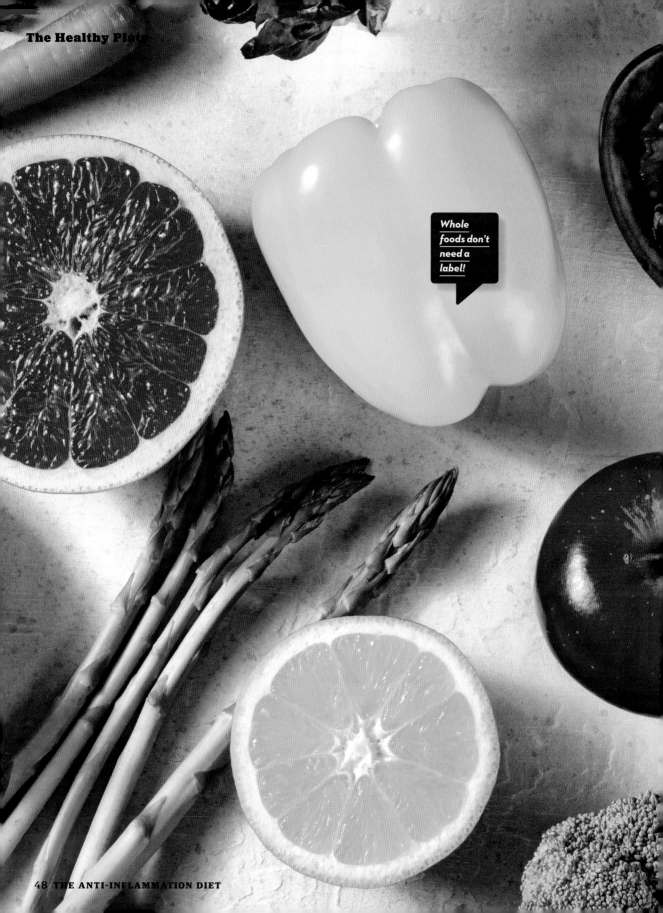

The Anti-Inflammatory Diet Plan

What you eat has a direct impact on your gut, heart, weight, blood vessels, brain and more.

Two of the healthiest eating plans for heart disease—the Mediterranean and the DASH (Dietary Approaches to Stop Hypertension) diets—also top the list when it comes to turning down the flame on inflammation. These plans emphasize whole foods, especially vegetables, fruits, legumes, nuts and seeds, and whole grains, as well as seafood and poultry that are low in saturated fat. The DASH diet is designed to increase the intake of nutrients such as potassium, calcium and magnesium—all good inflammation fighters—and reduce the intake of sodium.

"Diet is a foundational tool by which we can dial back inflammation," says Marzena Slater, MD, a physician at Root Functional Medicine in Grand Rapids, Michigan. And it's not just about the food. The lifestyle habits that surround the Mediterranean eating style—being social and feeling connected to your community, good sleep, being physically active and low stress—also help turn down inflammation.

Food and Your Gut

As you probably know by now, there are trillions of bacteria (and some viruses and fungi) living in your gut. They feed on the food you eat and the dietary mix you serve up will alter the various communities. A diet high in red meat, sugar and processed foods will cause unfavorable bacteria to get a foothold, while a diet high in healthy fiber and fat, vitamins and minerals and polyphenols from plants will keep the good bacteria thriving.

The ratio matters because the bacteria create metabolites, chemical compounds that basically drive many of your bodily processes. They send signals to your brain, heart, lungs, liver, reproductive tract and more, which affects their functioning in good or bad ways. With every bite you're sending a message to your body. You want that message to be clear and here's how you do it.

Inflammation Fighters

Fiber This nutrient makes the magic happen, not just in the bathroom but throughout your body. "All plants have

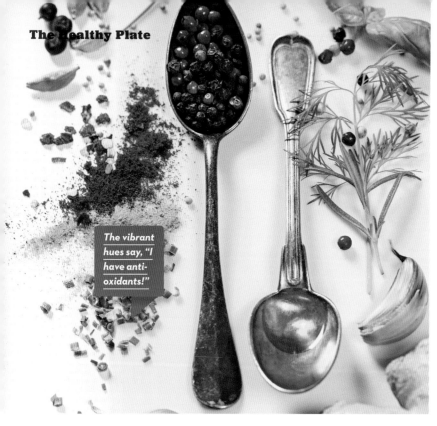

The vibrant hues say, "I have anti-oxidants!"

PEOPLE WHO EAT HIGH AMOUNTS OF FIBER LIVE LONGER LIVES.

Low Glycemic-Index Foods

The glycemic index (GI) is an indicator of how quickly sugar from food hits your bloodstream (table sugar has a GI of 100; an egg has a GI of 0). When that happens, insulin has to be released to shuttle it to cells.

But the GI index only goes so far. The glycemic load (GL) calculates a food's impact on your blood sugar based on the grams of carbs that you're eating. And that load is cumulative throughout the day. Here's the formula: glycemic load = (GI x grams

fiber so a plant-based diet is important," Slater says. "It slows absorption in the gut so you have a lower glycemic index (it won't spike blood sugar levels), it increases energy density and feeds healthy bacteria in the belly. As the bugs go to work fermenting fiber, they release short-chain fatty acids (SCFAs), which are anti-inflammatory for the colon."

Antioxidant-Rich Foods

While fruits and vegetables don't have a lock on antioxidants, they are your go-to source, especially because these little disease- and inflammation-fighting compounds come packaged with all sorts of other

good-for-you nutrients inherent in plants. "I do a 30-plant challenge for my clients," says Slater. "I encourage them to eat 30 different plant-based colors throughout the week, which is four to five servings a day."

Mediterranean at a Glance

DAILY
- ❏ Vegetables and fruit
- ❏ Whole grains
- ❏ Olive oil (limited portions)
- ❏ Beans/legumes
- ❏ Nuts and seeds
- ❏ Herbs and spices

TWICE A WEEK OR MORE
- ❏ Fish and seafood

WEEKLY
- ❏ Poultry, eggs, cheese and yogurt

SPARINGLY
- ❏ Meat and sweets

of carbs)/100. A cup of cooked oatmeal has 27 g of carbs and a GI of 55. That gives you a GL of 14.85.

You can reduce the glycemic load of a food by eating less of it, and you can reduce the total load you consume by eating fewer foods with carbohydrates. Low GL foods are those with a score of 10 or lower, medium are 11 to 19 and high are 20 or more. The goal is to keep your total daily GL below 100.

"We know that high glycemic load diets are associated with higher high-sensitivity C-reactive protein," says Slater. "Hyperglycemia can also create more oxidative stress in the body."

Omega-3 Fatty Acids These polyunsaturated fatty acids (aka PUFAs) are known for their anti-inflammatory effects. You can find the most easily absorbed kind in fatty fish and wild cod, says Sara Peternell, BCHN, a holistic nutritionist and owner of Family Nutrition Services in the Denver area. You can also find it in grass-fed beef. (Grain-fed beef has higher concentrations of omega-6 fatty acids, which Americans tend to overconsume.) Plant sources of omega-3s include walnuts and flaxseed, but the omega-3s in these foods are harder to absorb.

Fire Starters

REFINED SUGAR
Whether it's a soda, bottled juice or a sweet treat, sugar "has no nutritional benefit and it depletes the body's stores of magnesium, zinc and B vitamins," says Sara Peternell, BCHN. Excess sugar gets stored as fat, which creates inflammation, and a diet high in refined sugar can contribute to insulin resistance. Sugar-rich foods also bind with proteins and create compounds called advanced glycation end products (AGEs), which have been shown to trigger inflammation.

SATURATED FAT
While there's controversy over exactly how bad saturated fat is, so far the research reinforces limiting it in your diet. Saturated fat comes from animal products, including meat and dairy. A 2016 study in the journal Cell found that saturated fats "short-circuit" immune cells, leading to inflammation. Interestingly, a 2019 study published in BMC Public Health found that lifestyle habits that accompany saturated fat intake—such as exercise—may impact whether they trigger inflammation.

PROCESSED MEAT
Pepperoni and salami make for a yummy pizza but regular intake of these cured, salted or smoked meats, which are high in sat fat, can raise the risk of stomach cancer and also contribute to inflammation, courtesy of AGEs.

ALCOHOL
"Like sugar, it doesn't offer anything nutritionally—at 7 calories per gram—and it drains the body's nutrient reserves," Peternell says. "Plus, the liver and digestive system have to detoxify it and get it out of the body." The act of metabolizing alcohol creates inflammation.

PRESERVATIVES, CHEMICAL ADDITIVES AND ARTIFICIAL FLAVORINGS
"Your body knows what to do with a carrot or a chicken thigh. It doesn't know what to do with these," says Peternell. "They confuse and tax the body and create a permanent inflammatory situation." Spot them by reading labels and looking for food coloring and complicated ingredients, such as monosodium glutamate (MSG).

Healthy Fats While omega-3s are polyunsaturated, the kind of fat found in many nuts, seeds, olives and avocados is monounsaturated (aka MUFA). "It helps combat inflammation," Peternell says. "It's the fire extinguisher to put out the flame of inflammation and take the heat in the body down a notch. MUFAs inhibit inflammation in cells compared to saturated and trans fats, which turn it up."

Herbs and Spices These are highly condensed treasure troves of antioxidants and other nutrients. Think: turmeric, rosemary, ginger, basil, garlic, lavender. They add a whole extra layer of flavor and enjoyment to foods and combat rogue reactive oxygen species that trigger inflammation.

ID Your Triggers

Sometimes you may be eating the right things, but they're still not right for your body. "Food has many different components to it that can be a trigger for inflammation," says Peternell. "Most common is that certain proteins in foods can be antigenic, provoking an allergic reaction in the body. The immune system in the gut perceives that protein as a foreign invader and launches an inflammatory response."

People with food allergies have a reaction every time they eat a food, and it's possible to develop these allergies spontaneously as an adult. When you have a food allergy, the response happens within minutes as the body launches an assault. That could be nausea, diarrhea, hives or difficulty breathing.

The eight types of foods most likely to cause an allergic reaction are eggs, milk, peanuts, tree nuts, shellfish, fish, soy and wheat. An immunologist can do testing to determine whether you have a food allergy.

Then there are food intolerances and sensitivities, which are similar in nature. Intolerances are more serious sensitivities. These may take up to a few days to show up after you eat the food. "An intolerance originates in the gut or is primarily due to leaky gut, where those antigens are permeating the gut layer. As a result, the immune system reacts and goes after it," Peternell says. But that immune reaction is different

The Scary Thing About Celiac

It can be tricky enough to finally nail down a diagnosis of celiac disease, a condition where your body can't tolerate gluten, the protein found in grains such as barley, wheat and rye, and it starts attacking the lining of the small intestine. The condition can lurk, with mysterious and frustrating—or even mild or no—symptoms for years.

In addition to injuring the gut, celiac can also inhibit fertility, cause anemia, contribute to osteoporosis and more—thanks to the inhibited absorption of key nutrients. Having celiac disease also ups your risk of having another autoimmune condition. According to the Celiac Disease Foundation, if you have celiac, you have an 11% increased risk of developing multiple sclerosis, an up to 15% increased risk of Sjogren's syndrome and Type 1 diabetes, and a 5% risk of developing Hashimoto's thyroiditis, the leading cause of hypothyroidism. If you have these conditions and are having GI troubles, ask your doctor if you need to be screened for celiac.

from what happens with a food allergy.

Intolerances and sensitivities are harder to suss out with testing—many food tests have high false positive rates, leading people to cut out foods that may not actually be problematic. That's where an elimination diet comes in handy. "Food intolerances can come and go," Peternell says. "If you heal up the gut and do an elimination or rotation diet [to figure out what's triggering symptoms], it can help. You need to 'heal and seal' the gut."

Probably the most common intolerance or sensitivity is to gluten, which is a protein found in grains such as wheat, rye and barley. It turns out, gluten is a "gateway sensitivity." "To quote Italian gastroenterologist and researcher Alessio Fasano (who specializes in celiac disease and the spectrum of

CONCERNED YOU HAVE CELIAC? DON'T CUT OUT GLUTEN BEFORE GETTING TESTED.

DIET TIP An oral food challenge accurately tests for allergies.

gluten sensitivities), 'When in doubt get the gluten out!'" Peternell says. "When it comes to food intolerances, there's usually one or two, such as to gluten, gliadin (a protein within gluten), casein or whey (found in dairy) that will hold the door open [to other sensitivities] like a bouncer at a nightclub. If you get rid of gluten, you can get rid of other intolerances too."

You do that with a gluten-free diet. But cutting out wheat can limit your intake of otherwise healthy and nutrient-rich whole grains, so you have to be mindful to only cut out the offending varieties.

I Spy

If you're one of those people who has to be vigilant about what they eat—or else—it's time for a little investigative work. "My job is a lot like a private investigator, getting to the root of what's causing people to have struggles with their daily food choices," Peternell says. If you simply want to cut out inflammation in general, the Mediterranean diet is a good place to start. If you want to dig deeper, you can experiment with taking

certain foods out of your diet, such as dairy, gluten or sugar, and see how your body and brain react. To do a true elimination, where you take out potentially problematic foods and then add them back in slowly and in small amounts, it's best to work with a nutrition expert.

There are more restrictive diets for people with leaky gut or autoimmune issues. These include autoimmune protocol (AIP) diets and the GAPS (gut and psychology syndrome) diet. AIP diets are very restrictive and can be heavy on lean meat, seafood, vegetables, fruit and nuts, and oils from these items. They put the kibosh on dairy, legumes and grains, alcohol and, of course, anything processed or high in sugar. AIP diets also nix eggs and nightshades (tomatoes, potatoes, eggplant and peppers). Nightshades are high in healthy compounds, including some called glycoalkaloids, which certain people may be sensitive to.

The GAPS diet was developed for people with neurological or mental/emotional conditions, such as autism spectrum disorder and ADD/ADHD. The thinking is that what happens in the gut is affecting the brain. A certified GAPS practitioner can help you to navigate the different phases of the diet.

Bowled Over

We love a good plant-based recipe for delicious and satisfying meals that will fight inflammation at the same time—that's why you'll find more than 50 of them, starting on page 100. But sometimes you need something a little speedier, a go-to dish you can just pull out at the last minute. That's why bowls come in: They're a perfect, quick and healthy meal that you can customize any way you like with whatever you have on hand. Follow the lists to cover key categories (veggies, protein, whole grains, healthy fats) plus ways to amp up the flavor. It's an anti-inflammation dish that never gets old!

#2 Protein

The following will provide protein as well as fiber (if you incorporate beans). You only need about a half to three-quarters of a cup. If you really want to add meat, use it as a topping instead of the main protein.

- *Adzuki beans*
- *Black beans*
- *Cranberry beans*
- *Garbanzo beans (aka chickpeas)*
- *Lentils (red, green, brown, orange)*
- *Meat substitute*
- *Northern beans*
- *Red beans*
- *Tofu or edamame*

#3 Grains

These will provide healthy fiber and some even provide protein. Aim for whole grains versus white flour options. You only need about a half cup.

- *Amaranth*
- *Barley**
- *Brown or wild rice*
- *Farro**
- *Freekeh* (aka greenwheat)*
- *Israeli couscous**
- *Millet*
- *Quinoa*
- *Teff*
*Contains gluten

#1 Vegetables

Throw in all the veggies you want here (think: a cup or two). Roast or steam your veggies (you can do this ahead of time) or use them raw for extra crunch.

- *Arugula*
- *Avocado*
- *Beets*
- *Broccoli*
- *Broccolini*
- *Brussels sprouts (shredded)*
- *Cabbage*
- *Carrots (chopped small)*
- *Cauliflower*
- *Celery*
- *Green beans*
- *Kale (chopped small)*
- *Kimchi*
- *Kohlrabi*
- *Mushrooms*
- *Olives*
- *Onion (green, red)*
- *Peas*
- *Radishes*
- *Squash*
- *Sweet potatoes*
- *Watercress*

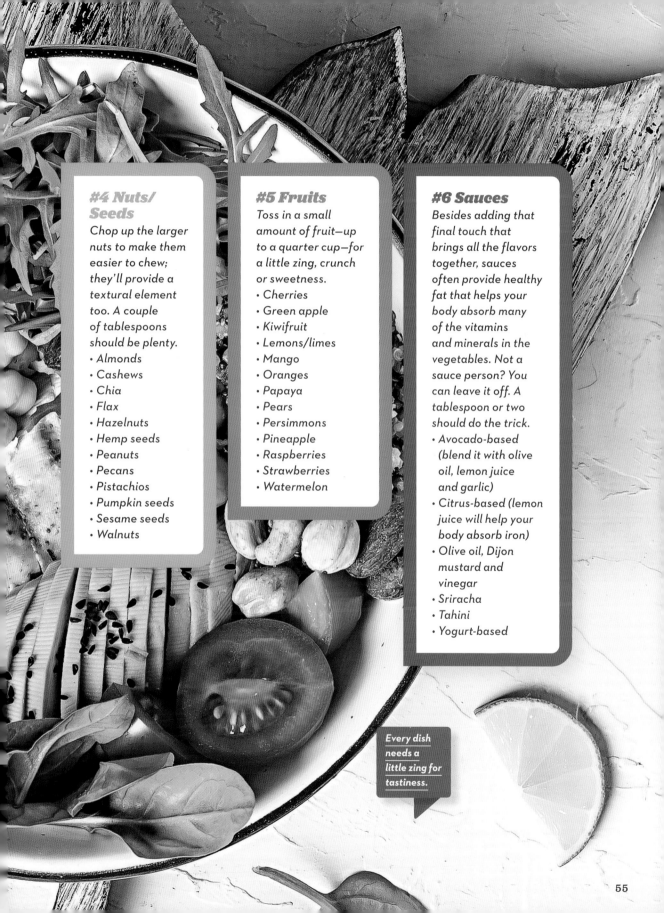

#4 Nuts/ Seeds

Chop up the larger nuts to make them easier to chew; they'll provide a textural element too. A couple of tablespoons should be plenty.

- Almonds
- Cashews
- Chia
- Flax
- Hazelnuts
- Hemp seeds
- Peanuts
- Pecans
- Pistachios
- Pumpkin seeds
- Sesame seeds
- Walnuts

#5 Fruits

Toss in a small amount of fruit—up to a quarter cup—for a little zing, crunch or sweetness.

- Cherries
- Green apple
- Kiwifruit
- Lemons/limes
- Mango
- Oranges
- Papaya
- Pears
- Persimmons
- Pineapple
- Raspberries
- Strawberries
- Watermelon

#6 Sauces

Besides adding that final touch that brings all the flavors together, sauces often provide healthy fat that helps your body absorb many of the vitamins and minerals in the vegetables. Not a sauce person? You can leave it off. A tablespoon or two should do the trick.

- Avocado-based (blend it with olive oil, lemon juice and garlic)
- Citrus-based (lemon juice will help your body absorb iron)
- Olive oil, Dijon mustard and vinegar
- Sriracha
- Tahini
- Yogurt-based

Every dish needs a little zing for tastiness.

Power Pairs

Taming inflammation starts on your plate, with healthy, delicious and gorgeous dishes. Food may be medicine, but that doesn't mean it has to be a bitter pill. These (mostly) classic duos will tempt your palate while also providing antioxidants, anti-inflammatory compounds and important vitamins and minerals. Medicine never looked so scrumptious!

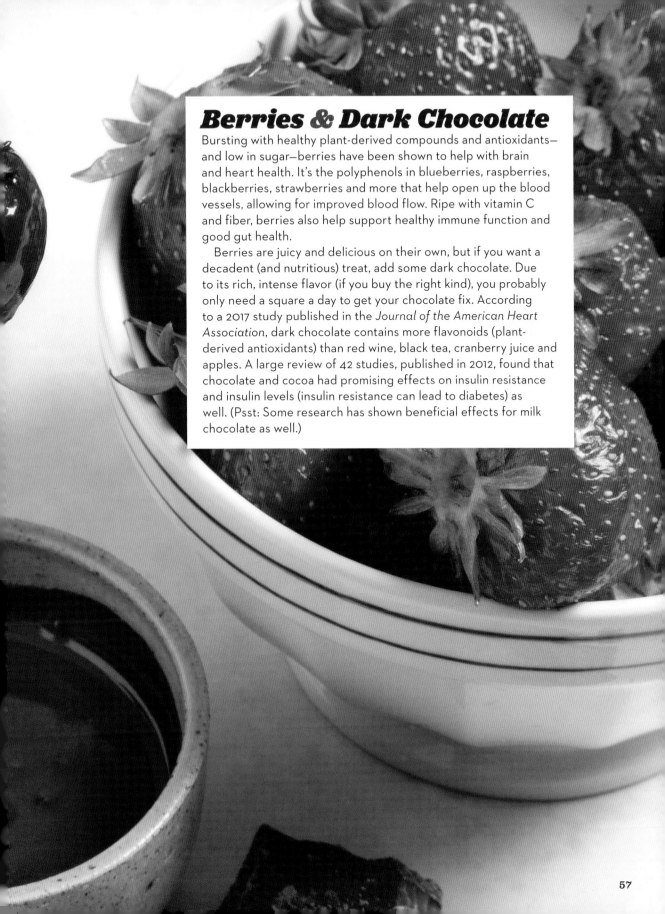

Berries & Dark Chocolate

Bursting with healthy plant-derived compounds and antioxidants—and low in sugar—berries have been shown to help with brain and heart health. It's the polyphenols in blueberries, raspberries, blackberries, strawberries and more that help open up the blood vessels, allowing for improved blood flow. Ripe with vitamin C and fiber, berries also help support healthy immune function and good gut health.

Berries are juicy and delicious on their own, but if you want a decadent (and nutritious) treat, add some dark chocolate. Due to its rich, intense flavor (if you buy the right kind), you probably only need a square a day to get your chocolate fix. According to a 2017 study published in the *Journal of the American Heart Association*, dark chocolate contains more flavonoids (plant-derived antioxidants) than red wine, black tea, cranberry juice and apples. A large review of 42 studies, published in 2012, found that chocolate and cocoa had promising effects on insulin resistance and insulin levels (insulin resistance can lead to diabetes) as well. (Psst: Some research has shown beneficial effects for milk chocolate as well.)

Turmeric & Bone Broth

Do any online searching and you'll see turmeric is synonymous with "anti-inflammatory." Thanks to its curcuminoids and volatile oils, the active chemicals in the spice that give it its vivid yellow-orange color—not to mention antioxidant capabilities—turmeric has been studied for all sorts of conditions that are linked with inflammation, including certain cancers, heart disease and Type 2 diabetes.

Take advantage of its benefits by adding a couple of teaspoons (and a pinch of black pepper to boost absorption) to freshly made bone broth. Savory and comforting, bone broth is rich in glutamine, a compound required for the health of your intestinal lining, as well as glycine and arginine, which have anti-inflammatory capabilities.

Feel free to add other healthy herbs and spices, including ginger, cinnamon and even cayenne pepper.

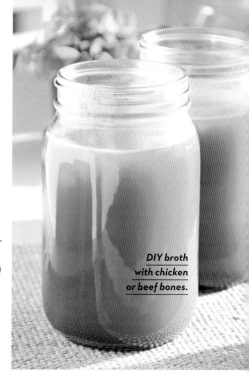

DIY broth with chicken or beef bones.

FAT IN BONE BROTH AIDS ABSORPTION OF TURMERIC, TOO.

Tuna & Avocado

Chefs have loved this combo for years (think: raw tuna poke tower with avocado and a touch of soy sauce), but this duo has legs even with packaged tuna. First, the fish is a good source of anti-inflammatory omega-3s, not to mention vitamins B12 and D. It also has other immune-enhancing compounds, such as vitamin C and selenium. (Look for canned light tuna to reduce mercury exposure and pole-and-line caught or troll-caught to reduce the ecological impact of tuna fishing.)

Now for that avocado. This darling of the food world adds creaminess to any dish—with a side of both healthy fat and fiber to boot. Monounsaturated fat targets inflammation in the heart and a compound called beta-sitosterol helps naturally lower cholesterol. Avocados are also a source of vitamin E, which is a powerful antioxidant.

Since both tuna and avocado are rich, you need a little zing to cut through the flavors; drizzle a little lemon or lime on top.

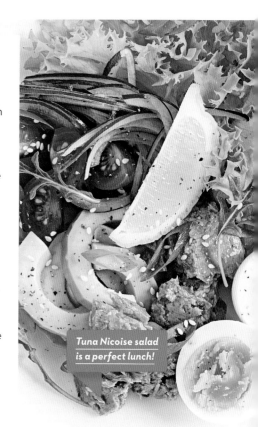

Tuna Nicoise salad is a perfect lunch!

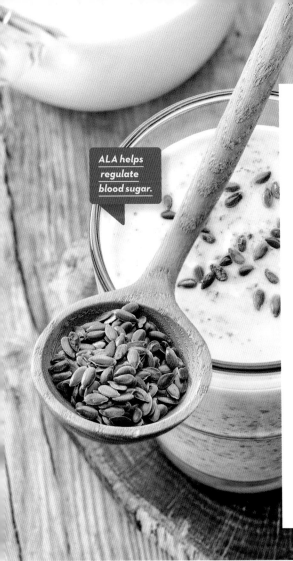

ALA helps regulate blood sugar.

Yogurt & Flaxseed

Yogurt contains healthy probiotics—live bugs that help populate your gut—and flax is an omega-3 rock star. Mix the two and you've elevated your breakfast. That cup of yogurt also contains calcium and protein, making it a satisfying meal that can keep you fuller longer. Look for low-sugar, plain Greek varieties and add your own berries or fruit to give it some natural fiber-rich sweetness.

Pop those flaxseeds in a grinder and sprinkle them over your yogurt to make the small, flat seeds easier to digest and more bioavailable. In just one tablespoon, you'll get a gut-friendly 2 grams of fiber and 2 grams of anti-inflammatory omega-3s, in the form of alpha-linolenic acid. FYI, a tablespoon of flaxseed oil, which you can easily use for dressings on veggies and is better absorbed than seeds, has triple the amount of alpha-linolenic acid (ALA).

If you're getting your omega-3s from plant sources, aim for 2.2 grams per day since your body has to convert it to EPA (eicosapentaenoic acid) and DHA (docosahexaenoic acid), the types found in fatty fish. High intakes of ALA are associated with a reduced risk of atherosclerosis, the buildup of fatty plaques in the arteries.

Salmon & Broccolini

A 2015 study published in *Nutrition Research* found that sulforaphane, a compound in cruciferous veggies such as cabbage, broccoli and Brussels sprouts (and so many more crunchy, delicious options), helps up-regulate selenium, a mineral that's important for immunity and keeping a lid on inflammation. (It's also beneficial for healthy, balanced thyroid function.) Broccolini also contains prebiotic dietary fiber, the kind that gut bugs like to munch on.

Salmon is also an omega-3 fatty acid all-star, boasting 1.2 grams of DHA in a 3-ounce serving, which is about half of the recommended daily dose of omega-3s (plus you're getting it with all sorts of other healthy nutrients as well).

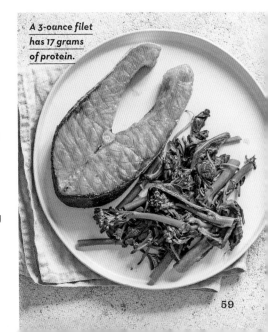

A 3-ounce filet has 17 grams of protein.

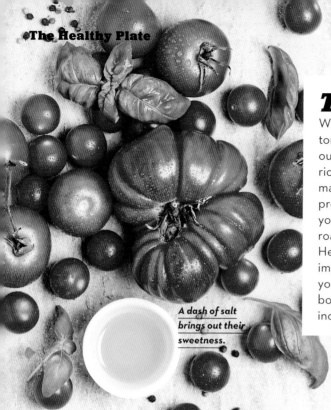

A dash of salt brings out their sweetness.

Tomatoes & Olive Oil

Who doesn't love olive oil drizzled on some juicy, ripe tomatoes? This classic summer combo never goes out of style. Among other nutrients, tomatoes are rich in lycopene, a polyphenol and antioxidant that may help prevent cancer, heart disease and other problems. But the key to unlocking the lycopene in your 'maters is to cook them, so lay them out on a roasting pan, grill them or turn them into a sauce. Here's the secret: Adding some olive oil will help improve absorption of lycopene. At the same time you'll be getting monounsaturated fat that your body uses for all sorts of important functions, including brain and heart health.

FIBER HELPS FIGHT INFLAMMATION IN THE GUT AND BLOOD VESSELS.

Beets & Chickpeas

Pairing these foods not only makes for a delish dip or topping, it's also gorgeous. Chickpeas (aka garbanzo beans) are off the charts in fiber: 17 grams in a half cup. They boost gut health by helping to feed good bacteria. A 2015 study of close to a million people, published in the *American Journal of Epidemiology*, found that people who ate the most fiber were almost 20% less likely to die during the 10-year study period compared to those who consumed lower amounts. Fiber is an inflammation scrubber, whether in the gut or blood vessels.

Beets, a classic root vegetable, are vascular powerhouses. Thanks to their nitrates (which raise nitric oxide), they help keep blood vessels open, reducing blood pressure and improving the flow.

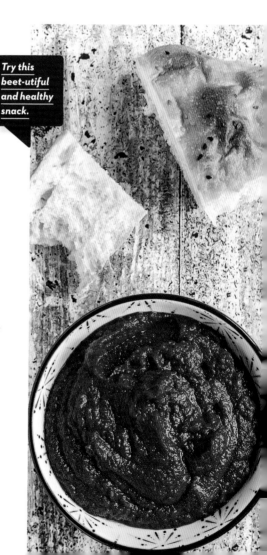

Try this beet-utiful and healthy snack.

Spice It Up

They're tiny but mighty. According to a 2019 study published in Genes & Nutrition, the most anti-inflammatory-rich spices include thyme, oregano, rosemary, sage, basil, mint, cinnamon, clove, lemongrass and nutmeg. In other words, each and every one is a winner.

CINNAMON *An insulin sensitizer, cinnamaldehyde, the active ingredient in cinnamon, has been studied in many trials. A 2013 analysis of 10 randomized, controlled trials found that regular cinnamon consumption (from 120 milligrams to 6 grams) for up to 18 weeks decreased blood sugar levels, "bad" (LDL) cholesterol levels and triglycerides in people with Type 2 diabetes. It may also increase HDL (good) cholesterol.*

MEXICAN OREGANO *Used to make chili powder and a staple in Mexican cuisine, this herb, which has more citrus notes than European oregano does (it's a different family), is high in cirsimaritin, an antioxidant and anti-inflammatory.*

ROSEMARY *Rich in carnosic and rosmarinic acids, two important polyphenols, rosemary is being studied for its anti-cancer properties, among other things. It grows easily indoors and out so you can harvest the spiky, aromatic leaves year-round for sauces, stews, rubs, sides and main dishes.*

SAGE *This herb lowers blood sugar and cholesterol and fights inflammation. In one study, steeping 4 grams of dried sage leaves in water and drinking it for two weeks reduced LDL cholesterol, among several other benefits.*

CAYENNE *This spice will heat up any dish but its active compounds—capsaicin and capsinoids—are used in topical creams as an anti-inflammatory to treat pain.*

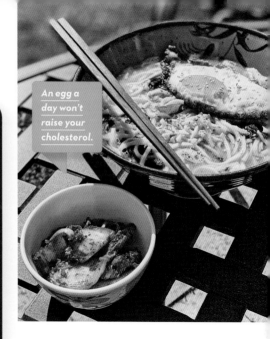

An egg a day won't raise your cholesterol.

Kimchi & Eggs

Chefs say everything is better with an egg on top, but we think the saying should be flipped: Everything, including eggs, is better with a little kimchi on top (or the side). This crunchy, spicy, tangy fermented cabbage (a Korean food staple) is a downright flavor explosion in your mouth. Due to the fermentation process that gives it the tang and extra heat, it's also good for your gut, providing healthy fiber and bugs to add to the good bacteria in your belly.

Eggs are little orbs of goodness too since they're loaded with omega-3s (if you buy the pasture-raised variety), vitamins and two key carotenoids—lutein and zeaxanthin—that have an anti-inflammatory effect in the eyes, protecting them from free radical damage.

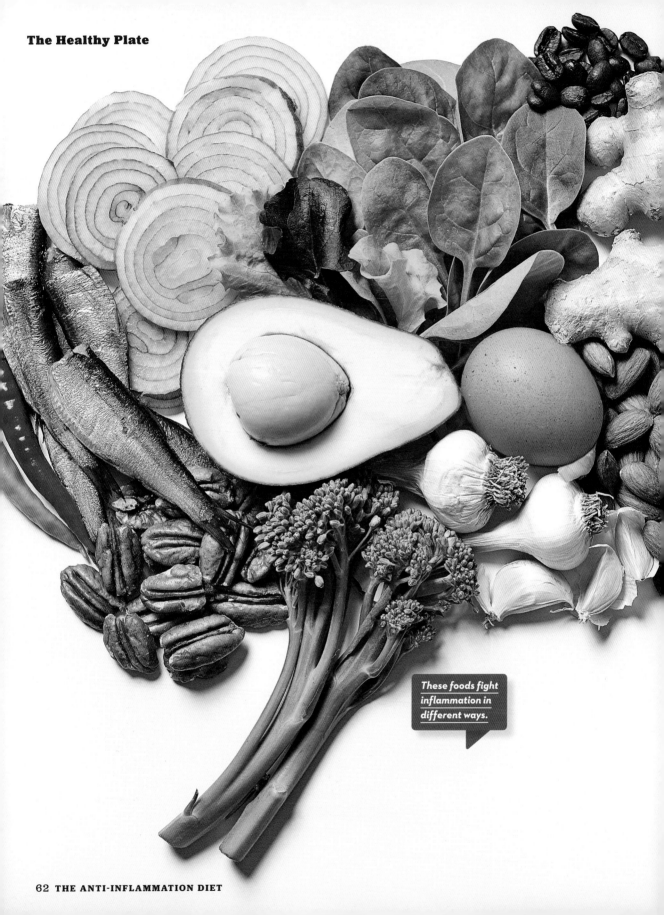

These foods fight inflammation in different ways.

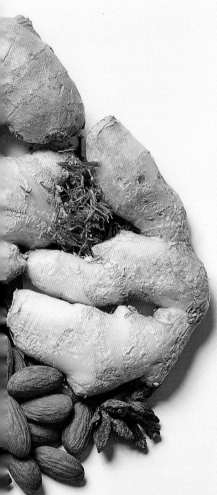

Everyone has the occasional brain "fart"—where you blank on info that's normally easily accessible—but sometimes that foggy, gauzy feeling in your head that makes it hard to focus or think clearly lingers. There are many potential causes, from stress and sleep troubles to medications and hormonal shifts, but there's one culprit that's easy to isolate and eradicate: your diet.

It's no secret that certain foods can affect your mood and mental acuity. "They call the gut the second brain. When your microbiome in your gut gets altered, it can affect your brain's production of neurotransmitters," says Rajsree Nambudripad, MD, an integrative medicine physician at Providence St. Jude Medical Center in Orange County, California. "Consuming anything that's inflammatory to your body will make you feel more agitated, irritable, anxious and depressed."

It doesn't take much either. One 2019 study investigating the link between inflammation and mental fogginess found that even mild inflammation in the body led study subjects to feel less alert.

Beat the brain drain with these
top noggin-nourishing foods that also
balance immune function.

Clear *the* Fog

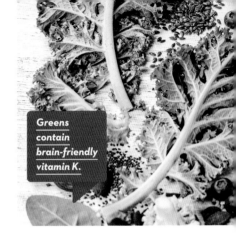

Greens contain brain-friendly vitamin K.

But that's not the only way your diet affects your noggin. Hypoglycemia—aka low blood sugar—can also be triggered by your eating habits. A diet too high in sugary carbs can lead to insulin resistance, which prompts an overproduction of insulin in an effort to overcome the cells' resistance to the hormone. That can tank blood sugar levels, leaving you feeling fuzzy brained, jittery, fatigued, "hangry" and more. If you frequently have those bouts, it's a sign that your blood sugars are having a hard time regulating, possibly due to insulin resistance.

Top Brain-Boosters

These five food superstars are the best for clearing your foggy head.

Eggs

Not only are eggs replete with vitamins such as B6, B12 and D, but the yolks contain a particular brain-boosting ingredient: choline. Never heard of it? You're not alone: In fact, this mighty nutrient

> **DIET TIP** *Intermittent fasting—large blocks without eating—may sharpen brain function.*

wasn't acknowledged by the Institute of Medicine as an essential nutrient until 1998, but it's since hogging the headlines as a regular star of studies, which note choline's impact on mental alertness and memory. "It's a precursor to acetylcholine, which is a neurotransmitter that controls your mood and memory," Nambudripad explains.

Nuts

Thank the magical combo of anti-inflammatory omega-3 fatty acids and polyphenols, plus lots of brain-boosting vitamin D, for nuts' good rep when it comes to mental functioning. "Walnuts in particular are great for the brain," Nambudripad says. "After all, they're even shaped like a brain."

Other noodle-nourishing nuts include almonds and hazelnuts, thanks to high vitamin E content (studies have linked it with better cognitive performance); almonds, which contain the brain-power compound phenylalanine; and cashews, which have copper and may increase oxygen flow to the brain.

Berries

Each color in fruits and vegetables gives us a slightly different nutritional makeup, thanks to their phytochemicals, chemical compounds created by plants to protect against bacteria and fungi. Scientists are just beginning to understand how these compounds affect human health, but research suggests they may have a protective effect against certain cancers. Berries have them to spare. "Phytochemicals are compounds our bodies don't necessarily *need*, but they enhance the health of the plant and if we eat them, they'll enhance our health, too," says Jenn LaVardera, RD, a Hamptons, New York-based dietitian at Naturipe Farms, a partnership of berry growers.

The berry-brain connection has been steadily researched since the 1990s, when the late neuroscientist James Joseph's blueberry study showed the brain-protective quality of antioxidants—which blueberries and other berries are rich in—thereby turning the little blue orb into an overnight sensation. Studies since have repeatedly shown the mental benefits of berries, and a little goes a long way too: One study found that women who ate just three servings of strawberries or blueberries a week delayed age-related memory decline. "I like this idea that just three cups a week helps, because it's not like you have to eat five cups a day to see a benefit," says LaVardera.

Tea and Coffee

Speaking of a little going a long way, drinking caffeine in moderation can also give your brain a boost. "As long as you're not caffeine-sensitive and get jittery from it, drinking one cup in the morning can help mental sharpness and clarity," says Nambudripad. One popular energy-boosting morning fix is bulletproof coffee, where you add butter and MCT oil (medium-chain triglycerides), which comes from coconut oil, to your java. Since fat is absorbed slowly, adding it to coffee adds an extra—and sustained—energy boost. (It's also higher in calories than a normal black coffee, thanks to the oil and butter.) "My patients tell me that it helps with their mental clarity," Nambudripad says.

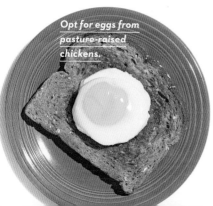

Opt for eggs from pasture-raised chickens.

What About Carbs?

No discussion about brain function is complete without delving into the topic of carbohydrates. "Carbohydrates are definitely the brain's preferred energy source," says Jenn LaVardera, RD. "The rest of the body can deal with fat or protein for energy, but the brain especially wants carbs." That's not a green light to stack your plate with pasta and bread, though, she adds. "It's easy to overdo it with carbohydrates, so half your calories should come from carbs and the other should be divvied up between protein and fat."

The type of carb you choose matters too, she adds. Stick with nutrient-dense options such as fruits, vegetables, legumes and whole grains to make sure you're getting important B vitamins, phytochemicals and fiber, and select foods that have a lower-glycemic index. "High-glycemic index carbs like pasta and breads can spike your blood sugar. That raises your production of insulin, which, if too high for too long, is inflammatory for the brain," says Rajsree Nambudripad, MD. "That's why I encourage patients to keep their meals balanced and have a blend of fiber-rich carbs, protein and good fats."

Just remember to adjust your caloric intake or you could end up gaining weight along with your clarity.

Leafy Green Vegetables

These nutrient powerhouses (think: spinach, kale, arugula and chard) are brain-friendly for two reasons, says Nambudripad. Their folate reduces gut inflammation and fiber helps feed good bacteria. One 2018 study showed that eating just one serving per day of leafy green vegetables (half a cup cooked, or one cup raw) is associated with slower age-related mental decline.

Nambudripad says cleaning up your diet can improve mental clarity, mood and energy—and gut health—in just a few weeks. Add these foods to your plate now and you'll be brain-fart-free soon.

Pick *Your* Pill

We scoured the supplement aisle and the research to uncover the best inflammation-fighters for a variety of conditions.

Inflammation manifests itself in a variety of ways and can be due to numerous triggers, including stress, trauma and, especially, diet. With more and more research pointing to the role it plays in fomenting disease, there's been an explosion of products that claim to fight the flame. It can seem a bit overwhelming, but the following supplements have undergone substantial research and come recommended by the experts who work with them every day.

Turmeric

You know that distinctive flavor and color in curry? It comes from turmeric (a relative of ginger), and it's earned superstar status for any number of things, including helping to reduce inflammation in people with Type 2 diabetes, inflammatory bowel disease and cancer. This is all thanks to its active ingredient: curcumin.

"Turmeric is particularly known to reduce inflammatory bowel-related inflammation, and it can also boost how easily absorbed certain medications are, so I always recommend that my patients try it," says Niket Sonpal, MD, gastroenterologist at Touro College of Osteopathic Medicine in New York City. You can use fresh or ground turmeric in foods or take it in capsules (research suggests at least 500 milligrams a day is ideal for fighting inflammation).

Probiotics

These help populate the communities of good bugs in your belly. They're alive in whole foods, such as yogurt and kefir, but they're also available in supplement form. Probiotics have been shown to be effective for a variety of conditions, including gastrointestinal and upper respiratory infections, atopic dermatitis and more. They may also help reduce inflammation in autoimmune conditions such as rheumatoid arthritis, ulcerative colitis and multiple sclerosis.

The strain you need will vary depending on the health issue you're dealing with. For overall gut health, you're better off looking for a product that contains a variety of probiotic strains and at least 10 billion colony-forming units (CFUs).

Wheatgrass

Besides containing vitamins A, C, E, iron, magnesium, calcium and amino acids, those bitter shots of green juice have inflammation-fighting cred. In one small study published in the *Scandinavian Journal of Gastroenterology,* just a half cup of wheatgrass juice daily for one month reduced inflammation symptoms in people with ulcerative colitis by 30%. Researchers believe the magic ingredient might be chlorophyll, a plant pigment with antioxidant powers.

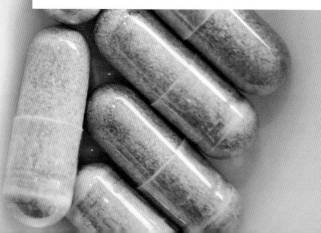

Use your supplements sparingly to reduce toxicity.

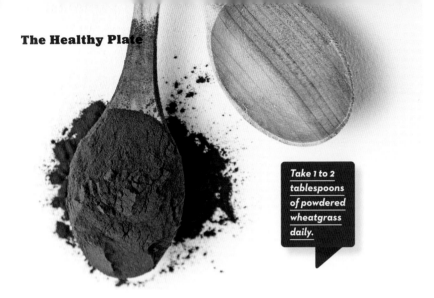

Take 1 to 2 tablespoons of powdered wheatgrass daily.

Fish Oil

While the research has been contradictory in terms of exactly which conditions omega-3s in supplement form (versus real food) can help treat, one thing most experts agree on is they have strong anti-inflammatory powers. "The omega-3 fatty acids that you get from fish oil supplements are vital to good health; they can decrease inflammation associated with diabetes, heart disease, cancer and many other conditions," says Sydney Spiewak, RD, a dietitian at Clinical Weight Loss & Wellness in East Hartford, Connecticut.

The main omega-3s are eicosapentaenoic acid (EPA), docosahexaenoic acid (DHA)—both of which are found in fish such as

SUPPLEMENT TIP
Look for the words "acid resistant" on the probiotic supplement label so you know it will make it through the stomach.

wild salmon, sardines and anchovies—and alpha-linolenic acid (ALA), which is found in walnuts and flaxseed.

Most research focuses on anywhere from 200 to 2,000 milligrams. Aim for 1,000 to 2,000 milligrams per day in a combo of DHA and EPA.

Vitamin C

This super-vitamin is renowned as an immune system protector and

antioxidant that can help eradicate the damage from free radicals. It also has anti-inflammatory powers: One 2015 study found that taking two 500 milligram doses of vitamin C a day helped people with diabetes- or hypertension-related inflammation reduce their levels of C-reactive protein, interleukin 6, fasting blood glucose and triglycerides. The recommended daily dose is 75 milligrams a day for women and 90 milligrams a day for men, but higher doses are well tolerated.

CoQ10

Coenzyme Q10 (aka ubiquinone or ubiquinol) has many functions, including protecting your cells from oxidative damage by neutralizing and minimizing damage from free radicals. It also boosts mitochondrial function (i.e., creates more energy). It's been used alone or with other drug therapies to prevent or treat heart disease and hypertension, periodontal disease, autoimmune issues, allergies, headaches and Parkinson's. A 2017 study in *PLOS One* found that supplementing with CoQ10 may help

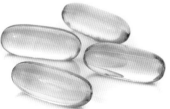

IF YOUR DIET IS LIGHT ON SEAFOOD, SUPPLEMENTING WITH OMEGA-3s CAN BRIDGE THE GAP.

THE SUPPLEMENT INDUSTRY WILL GROW TO $210 BILLION BY 2026.

improve the inflammation found in metabolic diseases, including obesity and diabetes. The standard dose ranges from 90 to 200 milligrams a day.

Vitamin D

This mighty vitamin, known best for building bones, is a key factor in immune system functioning. It not only boosts cells' ability to fight off and get rid of bad bacteria and viruses, it also helps regulate the immune response, pumping the brakes on an overactive response. People who are low or deficient in D may be more susceptible to chronic diseases, including those such as asthma,

Read Your Labels

Supplements are not regulated by the FDA (or anyone, for that matter), so you don't always know what you're getting. In 2015, the New York State Attorney General's office pulled a variety of herbal supplements—such as ginseng, St. John's Wort, echinacea and ginkgo biloba—from store shelves at major retailers because they didn't actually contain the ingredients that they touted. In fact, 79% of the products failed to contain any DNA from the product listed on the label!

That's where the USP-verified label comes in handy, says Sydney Spiewak, RD. "With it, you know you're getting what you see on the label, and that the product has met high standards," she says. The stamp also means the product is free of harmful levels of certain contaminants, such as pesticides, mercury and lead. (Learn more at usp.org/verification-services.)

No matter what you take, just remember to check in with your doctor. "Natural supplements can interact with medicines, so it's important to tell your doctor so they know everything you're taking, and can offer dosage recommendations," says Niket Sonpal, MD.

inflammatory bowel disease and kidney disease. It may even make you more susceptible to COVID. "If you're low in vitamin D, you can have more inflammation in your body and you won't be able to absorb calcium as well," explains Rajsree Nambudripad, MD, an integrative medicine physician at Providence St. Jude Medical Center in Orange County, California. The daily recommended dosage is 15 micrograms; 20 micrograms if you're over age 70.

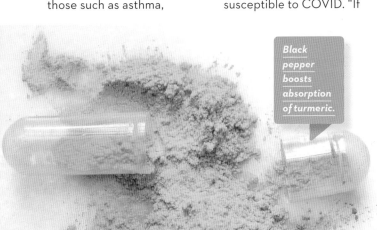

Black pepper boosts absorption of turmeric.

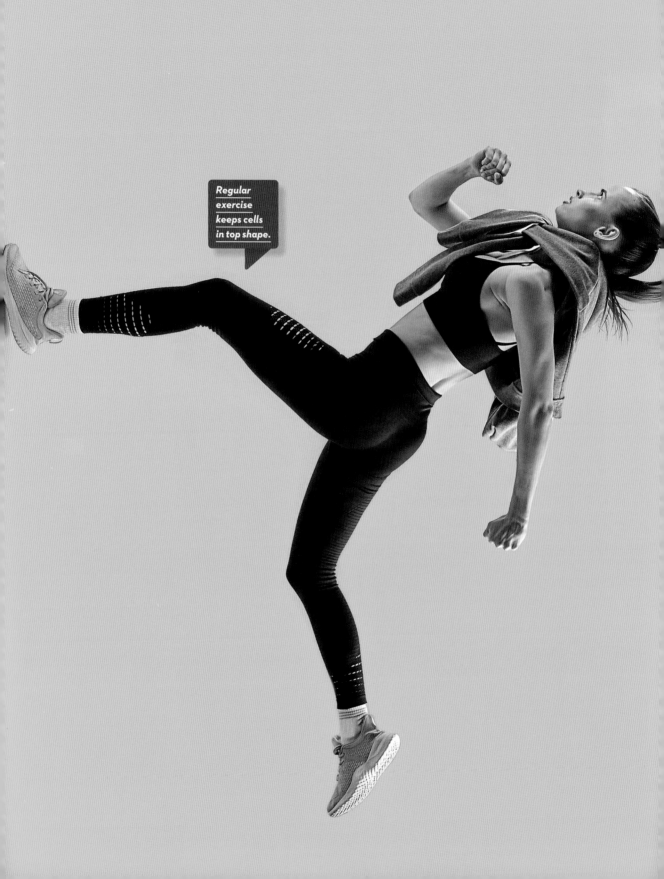

Chapter

3

Quell *the* Uproar

*Beyond diet, lifestyle habits
can help your body douse those
inflammatory signals.*

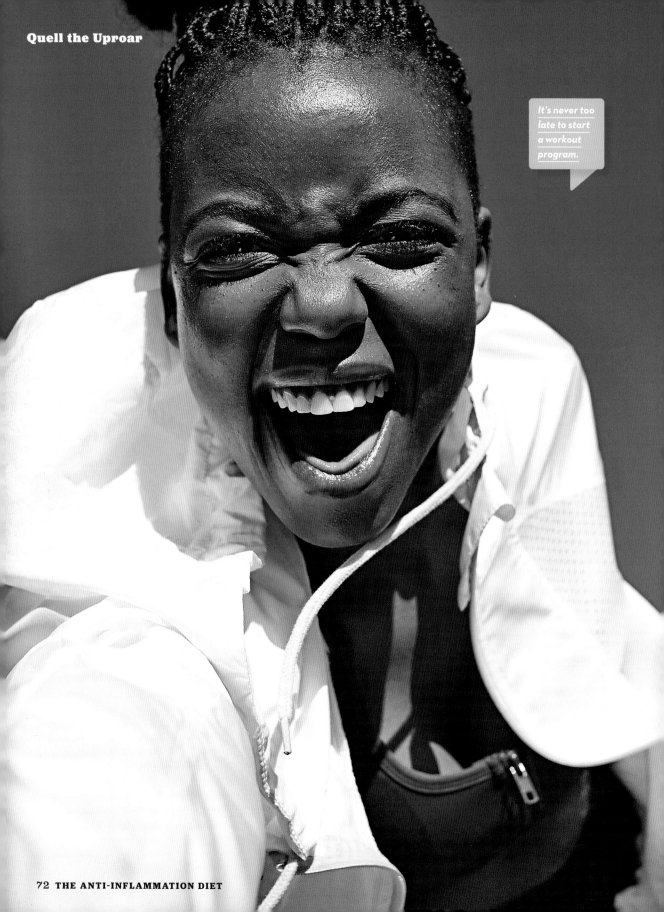

Why You Should ♥ Exercise

Working up a sweat helps reduce the risk of many chronic conditions, perhaps because of its effect on inflammation.

One of the most important things you can do to lower inflammation—and your risk of heart disease, obesity, diabetes, insulin resistance, cancer and more—is exercise. Getting your glisten on targets inflammation in a variety of ways, according to a large 2012 review of research published in *Aging and Disease*. The three main reasons: It reduces the accumulation of fat that can creep on with age (fat triggers inflammation), stimulates the parasympathetic nervous system, and triggers the release of your body's natural anti-inflammatory abilities. Exercise also makes it easier for your body to manage blood sugars and insulin, reduces cholesterol and blood pressure, eases depression and more.

If you're currently sedentary, any kind of activity is better than nothing and will have a positive impact on your health. You don't have to take up running; Whatever movement that makes your heart work a little harder will improve your fitness, and that boosts benefits even more. All it takes to start doing that is 30 minutes of activity a day on most days. "A half-hour of vigorous walking is a good 'dose,'" says Robert Harrington, MD, a Stanford, California-based interventional cardiologist and former president of the American Heart Association. "If you do more, it can create an incremental benefit for the heart, but that walk will give you a good base to start with."

Exercise is so powerful, the World Health Organization (WHO) has doubled down on the amount of aerobic exercise people should get. It now recommends everyone—even seniors and people with chronic diseases—accumulate 150 to 300 minutes of moderate intensity cardio exercise a week. If you add in vigorous exercise, you can get by with less, since every minute of vigorous exercise counts as two moderate minutes. In addition, you should do at least two strength-training workouts a week. (To get a sense of how that looks in a week, see page 76.)

Overpowering Benefits

This exercise time is so powerful, it can compensate for the negative health effects of too much sitting, which many of us have become all-too-accustomed to over recent years. (Sitting may trigger inflammation.) The authors of a 2020 review, published in the journal *Atherosclerosis*, concluded: "...high levels (60 to 75 minutes per day) of moderate-to-vigorous physical activity appear to eliminate the increased risk of CVD (cardiovascular disease) associated with excessive sedentary behavior. Replacing sedentary behavior with any intensity of physical activity will produce health benefits; however, the greatest benefits occur when replacing sedentary behavior with moderate-to-vigorous intensity physical activity."

FIT TIP It's time to add weight to a move if you can complete the upper end of your rep range (say, 12 reps) for two workouts in a row.

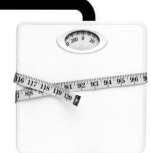

Should You Lose Weight?

Rates of obesity in the U.S. have been steadily rising for years. A 2017 National Center for Health Statistics report concluded that 43% of women and 38% of men over 60 are obese (a body mass index, or BMI, of 30 or higher). It's a big cause of inflammation (see page 28) and a contributor to other health conditions, including high blood pressure, nonalcoholic fatty liver disease and Type 2 diabetes. A 10-year study with more than 190,000 people (ages 20 to 79) found that being overweight or obese significantly increased the risk of heart disease and the issues associated with it.

But there's been some debate about how much a little extra weight affects your heart health, especially if you're older. An analysis in the American Journal of Clinical Nutrition *found that people 65 and older who had a BMI in the 27 to 29 range, considered "overweight," had the lowest mortality risk, compared to those with higher and lower BMIs. Other studies have shown similar findings. Extra weight may help protect against illness or falls and make you hardier if you have an illness or need to be hospitalized.*

Finally, researchers are exploring the link between the gut microbiome, inflammation and a tendency toward obesity. In the future, we may be able to target specific belly bacteria to avoid or correct that extra weight. For now, the fitter you are—at any weight—the better off you'll be.

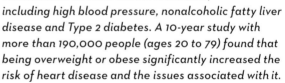

The large, randomized Look AHEAD (Action for Health in Diabetes) trial, which used exercise as part of an intense lifestyle intervention for people with Type 2 diabetes, found that those in the exercise group (they did 175 minutes a week) saw improvements in weight loss, fitness and blood sugar control and reduced blood pressure and cholesterol (along with a reduced need for medications) compared to the control group, which just got education with no intervention. The exercisers also saw a reduction in some of the most common side effects of diabetes, including kidney disease, sleep apnea, depression, sexual dysfunction, mobility, neuropathy and urinary problems. No single medication can even come close to accomplishing all that!

It's not just cardio that does a body good. Here's how other types of exercise benefit your health.

Be a Lean Machine

The WHO guidelines also recommend doing strength training—targeting your entire body—two or more times a week. Resistance training helps improve your body composition (the percentage of lean and fat tissue), bone mineral density, insulin sensitivity,

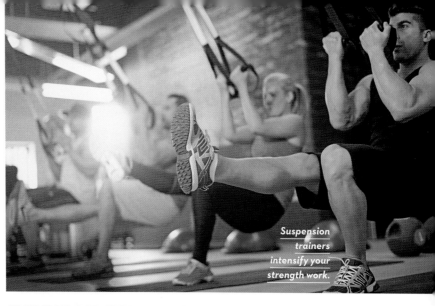

Suspension trainers intensify your strength work.

RESEARCH HAS SHOWN THAT STRETCHING MAY HELP LIMBER UP YOUR BLOOD VESSELS, TOO.

blood sugar control and cardiovascular risk factors. A 2019 study in *Medicine & Science in Sports & Exercise* found that people who did an hour of weight training each week had up to a 70% reduced risk of suffering a heart attack or stroke, compared to those who didn't lift weights. (Cardio exercise showed a similar benefit.)

Adding muscle has another protective effect, especially for people who are trying to lose weight (see sidebar on far left). First, lean muscle burns more calories per pound than fat does, so adding muscle increases the calories you burn at rest. When you start burning more calories than you're consuming, your body can tap into your muscles'

stores, which will slow your metabolism, making it harder to drop pounds. Maintaining or adding muscle as you lose pounds will keep your metabolism elevated and preserve strength that's crucial for staying mobile and avoiding falls.

While strength training does cause temporary inflammation in the muscles themselves, due to the fibers being broken down and then repaired, it's beneficial in the long run.

> **FIT TIP** At moderate intensity you can hold a conversation. At vigorous intensity you can only utter a few words at a time.

One Fit Week

Here's how to squeeze it all in.

SUNDAY *30-minute walk (cardio)*
MONDAY *30-minute strength-training circuit (strength + cardio)*
TUESDAY *45-minute walk (cardio)*
WEDNESDAY *30-minute HIIT session (cardio)*
THURSDAY *30-minute strength-training circuit (strength + cardio)*
FRIDAY *30-minute vigorous bike ride (cardio)*
SATURDAY *60-minute flowing yoga class (strength)*

Cardio = 135 minutes at moderate intensity plus 60 at vigorous intensity (counts double) = 255 minutes
Strength = 120 minutes

20-Minute Beginner HIIT Workout

MINUTES	EXERCISE	INTENSITY/RPE
0–5	Warm up	Light to moderate
5–5:15	Increase speed/resistance	Hard
5:15–6	Recover	Easy
6–11	Repeat minute 5 five times (alternating going hard for 15 seconds and recovering for 45 seconds)	Easy to hard
11–12	Maintain a moderate pace	Moderate
12–18	Repeat minute 5 six times	Easy to hard
18–20	Cool down	Easy

Add sprints between sets for a cardio burst.

A 2017 study in *Frontiers in Physiology* found weight training also had an effect on the immune system, helping balance the anti-inflammatory response and counteract the process of immunosenescence, age-related decreases in immune function.

Weight training doesn't mean grabbing barbells or jumping on bulky machines—although those are perfectly good tools if you're so inclined. Your own body weight may be sufficient to challenge your muscles, such as with squats, lunges, push-ups and core moves. There are also a ton of different aides out there to challenge your strength, including dumbbells, kettlebells and resistance tubes.

When strength training, hit each area of your body—legs, hips/glutes, abs, back, chest and arms—at least once a week, and aim for one to three sets of 10 to 15 reps, using a weight that's challenging by your final rep. Combine your strength moves with cardio to save time.

HIIT It Harder

Vigorous exercise—such as a speedy run, intense cycling class or super-steep hike—puts extra (good) stress on your heart and trains it to recover quickly. It can also improve how your body metabolizes fat and sugar and some research has shown high-intensity exercise targets visceral fat around your belly, which is highly inflammatory.

An easy way to work vigorous exercise into your routine is with high-intensity interval training, better known as HIIT. It's when you alternate going hard with easier recovery periods. "Hard" is relative, so anyone, at any level, can do it!

Adding in a couple of high-intensity workouts a week makes a significant dent in your exercise goals. The workout at left, which you can do with any type of cardio, starts with a short

EVEN CARDIAC REHAB PATIENTS CAN SAFELY DO INTERVAL TRAINING TO HELP BOOST FITNESS.

work interval and a longer recovery, which is on the easier end of the interval spectrum. Once you get the hang of it, you can make the work and rest intervals the same length and then start making your work periods longer than your rest.

Stretch It Out

Besides reducing stiffness and improving range of motion, stretching has two surprising benefits. First, it may help keep your blood vessels, which can become stiff due to atherosclerosis, more flexible. Second, it helps boost the body's natural anti-inflammatory responses, like for an injury. Activities such as yoga and tai chi, which also incorporate breathing and meditation, can help reduce stress while boosting flexibility.

Add five to 10 minutes of stretching post-workout to cool down, targeting all the areas of your body.

The Perks of a Workout Habit

- Reduces symptoms of depression and anxiety
- Helps prevent certain cancers
- Reduces the risk of heart disease
- Boosts cognition and learning ability
- Improves bone health and reduces the risk of falls
- Lowers the risk of stroke
- Reduces the risk of dementia

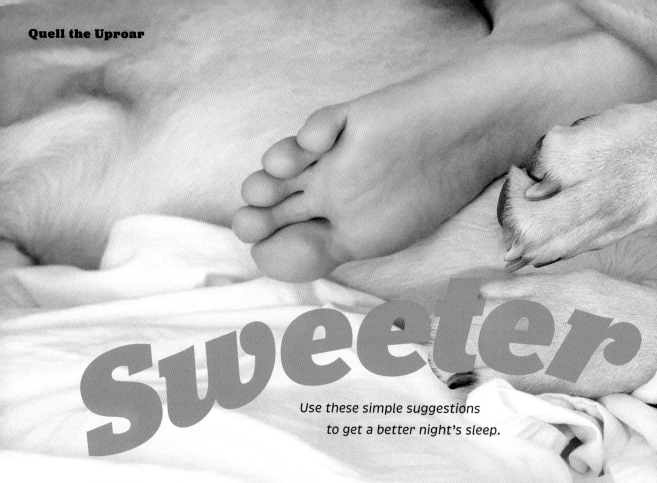

Sweeter

*Use these simple suggestions
to get a better night's sleep.*

Resting easy isn't quite so simple these days. More Americans are reporting getting worse sleep than before. Worry, isolation, feelings of depression and poor diet—which have all gone up in the past few years—can contribute to reduced snooze time. Put these all together and you have a recipe for increased levels of inflammation.

"Sleep is one of the key pillars of optimal health; it's just as important as the air we breathe and the food we eat. We spend a third of our lives sleeping and it directly affects the other two-thirds of our lives," says Mary Ellen Wells, PhD, an associate professor and director of the Neurodiagnostics and Sleep Science Program in the UNC Chapel Hill School of Medicine and UNC Charlotte in North Carolina. "On a biologic level, sleep has a mysterious restorative effect. Our brains are very active during sleep and they use a lot of energy. Research suggests the brain is doing some really important housekeeping work during sleep, consolidating memories and sweeping out the neural 'trash.' Levels of cerebrospinal fluid in the brain dramatically increase during sleep and it helps wash away the toxins that build up during the day."

Sleep and immune function are also directly related. Good sleep primes your body for daily activities and keeps your immune system functioning like it should, according to a review in the journal *Nature Reviews Immunology*. Lack of or disturbed sleep, in turn, "contributes to the dysregulation of inflammatory and antiviral responses," according to the review's author.

Whatever is keeping you awake, there are a few

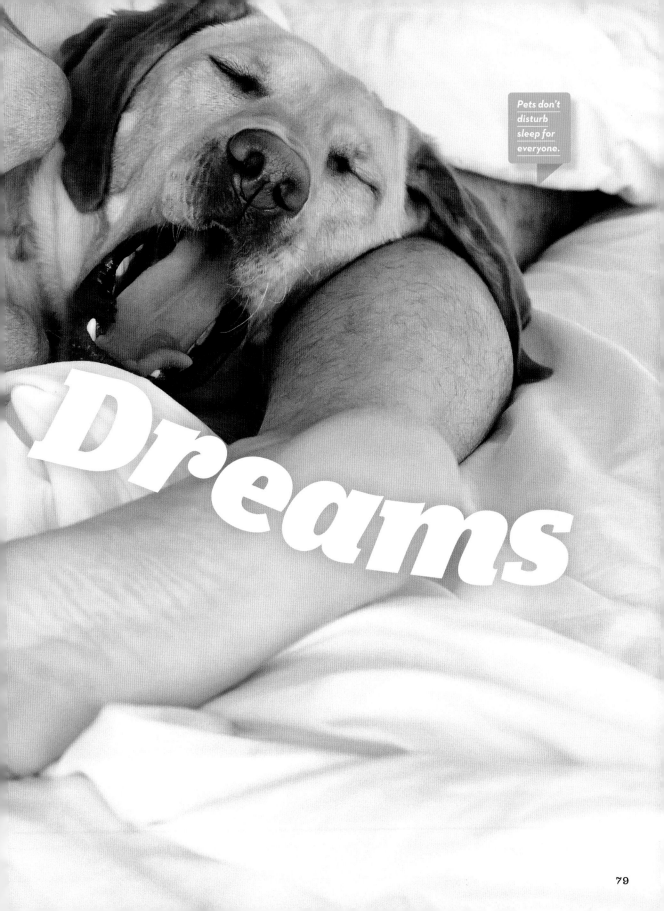

Pets don't disturb sleep for everyone.

Dreams

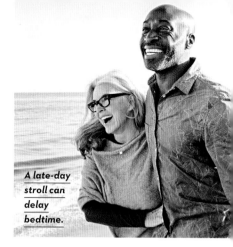

A late-day stroll can delay bedtime.

key areas where you can make changes and see big payoffs. Start by making sleep a priority, which means choosing it over other activities, carving out time and making it easy to switch into sleep mode. These daily habits will make it easier to go dark.

Make It a Priority

So many people bemoan their sleep deficit yet can't bring themselves to cut their binge-watching short. (Much like how you opt for happy hour over a sweaty cycling class.) Identify your eight-hour mark and start setting the stage an hour or so before that so when the time comes, you're pulling up the covers and turning off the light.

Be Consistent

Sleep experts are adamant in their recommendations around routine—and not just getting your typical allotment of z's. If you're an eight-hour-a-night person, you're better off maintaining a set sleep-wake schedule—say, going to bed at 10 and getting up at 6—than just trying to get

> **SLUMBER TIP** *Need fewer z's? Stick with your same sleep time frame—say, 11 to 7—as usual, even if it's shorter.*

your eight hours at any time. That means you shouldn't go to bed at 10 p.m. one night and midnight at another. You can still feel and function as if you're sleep-deprived if you get those eight hours but at a different time. Your brain and body like a schedule, in other words. The more you can stick to it, the better your *entire* body will run, including your immune system and GI tract, which also work on a schedule.

That doesn't mean you'll always need eight hours of sleep. As you get older, sometimes people find they need less snoozing time to function at their best.

Let There Be Light

Getting bright light early in the day is extremely important in helping to train your sleep cycle. When you're exposed to bright light later in the day or at night, like when you're staring at a screen a few inches from your face, it suppresses melatonin, the main sleep hormone, in the brain. (That late-day light exposure can help if you find you're having the urge to go to bed and wake up too early.) Morning daylight signals the brain, "Hey, it's daytime, see?" If you're inside all day, your brain doesn't get a clear signal and those natural tendencies start to dull.

Exercise Regularly

Daytime activities matter when it comes to prepping your body and brain for bed. All the things you do before getting into bed make a difference, including exercise. Working up a sweat, whether it's doing cardio, strength training or taking a yoga class, helps improve all your bodily systems—including squelching inflammation—and the healthier you are, the less likely you are to experience problems like sleep apnea or to be taking medications that might keep you awake at night.

Studies have shown that exercise helps make it easier to fall asleep and get better quality sleep and reduces the number of episodes of sleep apnea. Just time exercise no sooner than two hours before bed so it won't interfere with your z's.

Keep Work Separate

Raise your hand if you work from home—and you've spent the better part of your day in pajamas (or at least pajamas on the bottom) and in your bed, or both. Something as simple as putting on "daytime" clothes or moving to another room of the house gives your brain cues about sleep and wake time. When it's time for bed, establish your sleepy-time routine by dimming the lights, turning down the thermostat, getting into your sleep "uniform," and doing some calming breathing or gentle stretching. All these things signal the brain that z's are imminent.

Make a Healthier Plate

Research has shown that eating an anti-inflammatory Mediterranean-style diet may help you fall asleep faster and stay asleep. People who ate more legumes, fruits and vegetables, fiber, healthy fat and plant protein saw improved sleep.

Naturally, you shouldn't down a big meal right before bed since that can cause reflux or disturbed sleep. Plus, your body isn't timed to digest at 1 a.m. and the result could be increases in blood sugar, insulin resistance and cholesterol levels—or just more weight.

On the other hand, hunger can wake you up, so you may need to find the right snack timing pre-bedtime to ensure you're not awakened by a rumbling tummy.

Some people find they do better with a light snack before bed, such as chamomile tea, warm milk or fruit. The benefit of these has more to do with establishing a routine, than with any sleep-inducing benefits inherent in the food.

Customize Your Routine

Do you like a warmer room versus a cooler one? Then keep it warmer, as long as it's not disturbing your slumber. Prefer being surrounded by animals? Load them on. One study found that while 20% of sleepers said their pets disrupted their sleep, 40% said they made it better. The sleep "rules" don't apply to everyone. Pay attention to what's working (or not) for you and go from there.

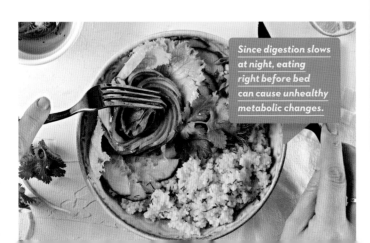

Since digestion slows at night, eating right before bed can cause unhealthy metabolic changes.

Should You Take These Drugs?

Anti-inflammatories can cause more trouble than they're worth. Here's what you need to know.

NSAIDs MAY INCREASE HbA1c LEVELS IN PEOPLE WITH DIABETES.

Whether it's a sprained ankle, period pain, arthritis or a fever, one of the quickest ways to tackle acute inflammation is with an over-the-counter anti-inflammatory, usually something called a non-steroidal anti-inflammatory drug, or NSAID. These include aspirin as well as naproxen (Aleve) and ibuprofen (Advil, Motrin). In the U.S., people take more than 30 billion doses of NSAIDs each year, with 15% of the population downing them regularly.

While they can be incredibly effective, in most cases, anti-inflammatory medications don't come without side effects, including stomach ulcers and bleeding, heart attack risk, liver failure (in the case of acetaminophen, which is not an NSAID) and more. It just goes to show that fighting inflammation is a complicated process that has implications throughout the body. All the more reason to know the pros and cons of your OTC anti-inflammatory of choice.

NSAIDs

These drugs work by inhibiting enzymes called COX-1 and COX-2 that are responsible for producing prostaglandins, a natural compound that the body releases at the first sign of an injury or infection. They're like little red flags that send up all the signals of inflammation, including pain, swelling and fever. COX inhibitors block the prostaglandin-producing enzymes to reduce inflammation, pain and fever. Some NSAIDs block both COX-1 and COX-2, while others just block COX-2.

Since prostaglandins can have a beneficial role in the gut, blocking both types of enzymes raises the risk for stomach upset and ulcers. "NSAIDs are more problematic [than other pain relievers] for GI upset and gut health," says Shabnam Sarker, MD, a gastroenterologist at Vanderbilt University Medical Center in Nashville, Tennessee. "They cause gastritis, or inflammation of the GI tract, especially in the stomach, because they block

prostaglandins, which is this chemical that protects your stomach lining and helps you create mucus. So when you take NSAIDs, it can be more pro-inflammatory. And then the medication itself can also be directly irritating if it's sitting in your stomach. That's why pharmacists usually tell you to take it with food, to protect the lining."

Research has shown that NSAID users have a different microbial composition than nonusers. The long-term impact of altering the microbiome is largely unknown, but an imbalance can cause abdominal discomfort, bloating or

More than 500 medicines contain acetaminophen.

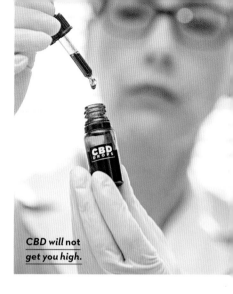

CBD will not get you high.

even affect the body's ability to absorb nutrients.

Within just 12 to 24 hours after taking an NSAID, intestinal permeability is increased. This means that the intestinal lining becomes looser and more vulnerable, allowing for bacteria and toxins to escape into the bloodstream, causing inflammation. This is commonly referred to as "leaky gut," although it's not well understood or easily diagnosed given the many factors affecting the GI tract. Still, the inflammation it causes is thought to contribute to myriad health problems, some chronic.

Besides potential gut-related issues, NSAIDs—with the exception of aspirin—also increase the risk of heart attack and stroke, especially when you first start taking them.

Three of the most popular NSAIDs you can find over the counter are ibuprofen, naproxen and aspirin. *Ibuprofen* is commonly used to reduce general inflammation (toothache,

fever, muscle aches) and pain, usually working within 20 to 30 minutes. It can be hard to tolerate on an empty stomach and the most common side effects are diarrhea, vomiting, nausea or abdominal pain. NSAID users older than 60, heavy drinkers (more than three drinks a day) or drug users are at

CBD RAISES LEVELS OF A COMPOUND IN THE BODY THAT REGULATES IMMUNE FUNCTION, PAIN AND MORE.

higher risk of experiencing stomach bleeding. *Naproxen* works similarly to ibuprofen to help counter inflammation, but it provides longer-lasting relief— typically up to 12 hours versus four hours.

In animal studies, taking naproxen orally, even for a short period of time, changed the gut microbiota composition and caused intestinal inflammation and ulceration. Some other side effects may include stomach pain, constipation, diarrhea, gas, vomiting, heartburn or dizziness.
Aspirin is known for its fever-reducing and blood-thinning effects. While all NSAIDs slow clotting to some degree, aspirin has a stronger effect.

Many people take baby aspirin (81 milligrams) as a preventive blood thinner for heart problems (always speak with your doctor about this first).

Aspirin has a bad rep for causing stomach upset or bleeding, but "if your primary care provider or cardiologist feels that you need to be on aspirin, the heart trumps the GI tract; take aspirin if you need to," says Sarker.

Other Options
Acetaminophen, the active ingredient in Tylenol, is a pain reliever and fever reducer (both signs of inflammation) but it's not technically an anti-inflammatory—and researchers are still trying to figure out exactly how it works. It's good for pain,

> **DOSING TIP** More isn't better! If you're taking one product with NSAIDs or acetaminophen, don't add another one.

headaches or if you have a bad cold with fever. It won't cause stomach upset, a bonus if you have nausea and vomiting with cold symptoms. But it does affect your liver. According to the Mayo Clinic, overdosing on acetaminophen—which is easy to do since so many products contain it—is the most common cause of acute liver failure in the U.S. You shouldn't take it with alcohol or if you're a heavy drinker (three or more drinks a day).

"Acetaminophen takes a different pathway than NSAIDs do," says Sarker. "People who have inflammation of their colon or stomach should probably avoid NSAIDs in general and try something like acetaminophen or a different type of agent."

CBD (aka cannabidiol), a non-psychoactive compound derived from the hemp plant, shows promise for regulating chronic or acute pain. While it doesn't work through the same mechanism as NSAIDs, it does affect how the immune system responds to inflammation. More research is needed to determine the full spectrum of conditions that CBD can help with. If you're looking for an alternative to NSAIDs, ask your doctor about CBD (or options with THC in states where it's legal).

Getting to the Root

Treating the underlying cause of the inflammation, of course, can help you avoid the negative side effects and risks of NSAIDs. "If you're using NSAIDs regularly, or if you're getting GI upset, then we really need to think about alternatives," Sarker says, "and also figure out what's causing that chronic pain or inflammation."

As with any drug, it's important to take the lowest dose that's still effective and for the shortest time possible. Then monitor your reaction and any side effects. If you find that you still need pain relievers or anti-inflammatories past the recommended time span on the bottle, talk to your doctor.

The Big Guns

Chronic inflammation can last for years, but, unlike acute inflammation that's an important part of the healing process, chronic inflammation has no purpose. When you have lingering pain, swelling, low-grade fever or other problems and OTC drugs aren't helping relieve your symptoms, your doctor may prescribe a corticosteroid—aka a steroid.

These drugs mimic cortisol, a hormone produced by the adrenal glands. While cortisol is better known as the "stress hormone," it's actually a very potent anti-inflammatory hormone that reduces the tissue and nerve damage caused by inflammation.

People living with inflammatory conditions such as rheumatoid arthritis or those suffering from acute pain related to a musculoskeletal problem (think: sciatica) can benefit from steroids. Cortisone, prednisone and methylprednisolone are some of the steroids prescribed for chronic illness or autoimmune disorders, where the body's immune system has turned on itself. They reduce inflammation by lowering the activity of the immune system. Drugs like these can be lifesaving as they reduce inflammation that could do lasting damage to tissues and organs. But beware: Since they also suppress the immune response, long-term use can increase the risk of infection.

A Toothy Topic

The connection between gum disease and heart disease is clear: It's all about inflammation.

Unlike in Vegas, what happens in the mouth doesn't stay in the mouth. Gum disease increases your risk of heart disease by 20% or more and significantly raises your risk of heart attack, according to a 2016 study in the journal *Circulation*. Inflammation is the common denominator—and it doesn't stop at the heart. Some research suggests there's a link between gum disease and other systemic conditions as well. All the more reason to brush and floss daily and see your dentist regularly.

A Slow Burn

Also called periodontitis or periodontal disease, gum disease is like a fire. It starts with a spark and, if not extinguished, can become an inferno. Sound familiar? The spark is plaque, a sticky film that naturally forms on teeth when harmless bacteria that's normally present in the mouth interacts with sugars and starches from foods we eat. If you don't brush well and regularly, the plaque can turn into tartar on the gumline. This hard buildup is difficult to remove but dentists can get rid of it during professional cleanings.

If you fail to see a dentist and the tartar accumulates, you can develop gingivitis. This mild form of gum disease causes inflammation and irritation around the base of the teeth. Left untreated, it can grow into periodontitis: The inflammation worsens and the gums become infected and damaged, which can even cause loose teeth or tooth loss if not treated.

The Road to Everywhere

But periodontal disease doesn't only affect your gums and teeth. "Our mouths are the gateway to our overall health. What's going on in your mouth can also affect other parts of your body— and sometimes in major ways," says Sanda Moldovan, DDS, a Los Angeles dentist and periodontist. "Every time gingival bleeding occurs, it presents an opportunity for microorganisms to enter the

Healthy gums should be firm and pink.

DAILY FLOSSING AND BRUSHING KEEP NORMAL BACTERIA FROM GETTING OUT OF CONTROL.

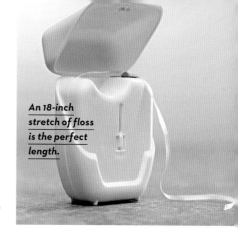

An 18-inch stretch of floss is the perfect length.

bloodstream and find a new home somewhere else, such as the joints, brain, lungs, blood vessel walls or placenta."

A growing body of evidence suggests a link between gum disease and other conditions, such as cardiovascular disease, gastrointestinal and colorectal cancer, diabetes and insulin resistance, and Alzheimer's disease, according to a study published in *Biomedical Journal* in 2019. Researchers and dentists have a few different theories about why these varied problems may be related.

One theory is that pathogens in the mouth trigger the immune system to kick into action in the mouth as well as in other areas of the body, leading to systemic inflammation.

Another theory has to do with the fact that gum disease causes pockets to form between your teeth and gums. As the disease worsens, these fill with more and more bacteria and the pockets develop sores. These sores may provide a door

for periodontal bacteria to directly enter your circulatory system. As the bacteria travel, they affect various organs and could lead to disease.

In the case of heart disease, heart attack and stroke, both of the above mechanisms seem to be at work: The bacteria from the mouth travel via the blood to the heart, where they damage the valves. Additionally, systemic inflammation from any cause increases the risk of heart problems.

Spot the Spark

The first way to protect yourself against any of these problems is to be aware of possible gum disease. Symptoms include:

> **Gums that bleed easily**
> **Gums that feel tender when touched or brushed**
> **Bad breath**
> **Red and/or swollen gums**
> **Pain when chewing**
> **Loose teeth**

Prevent the Fire

The best way to avoid gum disease—and possibly these other diseases—is likely what you're already doing: Take care of your teeth and see your dentist, especially if you notice any of the above problems. People who report brushing less than twice a day or for less than two minutes are three times more

likely to have gum disease compared to those who say they brush at least twice daily for at least two minutes, according to a 2018 study in the journal *Circulation*.

Then, seeing your dentist for a professional cleaning at least once a year lowers

HEALTHY TIP Polish your pearlies with an electric toothbrush, which is better at cleaning teeth than the manual-powered kind.

your risk of heart attack by 24% and your risk of stroke by 13%, compared to people who don't have regular cleanings, researchers reported in a 2012 study in the *American Journal of Medicine*. Going more often provides more protection.

Beyond oral hygiene, try to limit your intake of added sugars. "Excessive consumption of sugar is the number one enemy of achieving optimum oral

Your doc can also check for oral cancer.

health," Moldovan says. "After consuming sugary foods or drinks, rinse your mouth out with water if you're not able to brush your teeth."

Lastly, refrain from smoking or chewing tobacco. Both of these will weaken the immune system, making it harder for you to fight off any potential infection that may occur anywhere in your body, including in your mouth.

The Devil's in the Dental Work?

Holistic medicine is super popular these days and, as a result, holistic dentistry is becoming better known. Holistic dentists have dental degrees and treat the same conditions as traditional dentists. But holistic dentists consider how oral health impacts overall health and vice versa. They often point to dental work as the root of unseen inflammation. For example, many believe you cannot remove all bacteria during a root canal, which is when your dentist cleans out the infected nerve inside the roots and either puts in a filling or replaces the tooth with a crown. Holistic dentists believe lingering bacteria cause inflammation throughout the mouth and body. In some cases they'll remove crowns and extract the tooth completely. (Less invasive alternatives to root canals are being developed and extraction isn't recommended by traditional dentists unless a tooth can't be saved.)

The concern about rogue bacteria dates back to a flawed 1920s study stating that root canals led to arthritis, heart disease and other illnesses. That study was discredited in the 1950s, and evidence today doesn't support the idea that root canals or any other conventional dental procedures trigger inflammation. In fact, endodontic treatments, including root canals, are 86% to 98% successful.

According to the American Association of Endodontists, no valid, scientific evidence links root canals to health problems. If you're concerned, talk with your dentist about the best option for you.

Extinguish the Flame

If, despite your best efforts, you develop periodontal disease, don't panic. "Managing it at an early stage can lessen the risks of a number of illnesses in the entire body," Moldovan says. That's why it's so important to see your dentist at least once a year so they can check your gums.

The best way to treat gum disease is to remove the bacteria, says Neil Karnofsky, DDS, a periodontist in New York City and chief dental officer of ProHEALTH Dental. For minor cases, your dentist may do a deep cleaning (called scaling) to remove tartar and bacteria, prescribe topical or oral antibiotics, or perform root planing. This is when they smooth out the roots of your teeth, which helps the gums reattach to the teeth, preventing the buildup of more bacteria.

If this doesn't work or your disease is more advanced, you may need surgery, which is performed by a periodontist. Procedures include lifting a section of gum tissue to allow for deep scaling and root planing, recontouring the bone supporting your teeth so it's easier to clean them, and reinforcing receding gums.

Brushing regularly is sounding better, right? It's worth it to save your smile—and the rest of your health.

Stressors
affect
everyone
differently.

Stress Case

All that tension and aggravation can cause negative hormonal and immune system shifts, which puts you at greater risk of many common diseases.

Your nervous system doesn't care if you're being chased by a rabid bobcat or you're freaking out about a work presentation—the physiological response will be the same. Your body goes into survival mode, led by the sympathetic nervous system. Heart rate and blood pressure increase and the pupils dilate, so you can see any threats coming at you. This response also shuts down major bodily processes, such as digestion, reproduction and the immune system—because if you're about to be eaten by a wild animal, it doesn't matter if you come down with a case of the sniffles. "Your body is focused on the one imminent threat," explains Leah Owen, MC, LAC, an integrative psychotherapist based in Mesa, Arizona.

"However, this response is less useful in a chronically stressful environment like a high-pressure job, where the body just keeps pumping out stress hormones like norepinephrine, cortisol and adrenaline. You're going to get chronic health problems."

Stress and Inflammation

As soon as that imminent threat has passed, the parasympathetic nervous system is supposed to take over, calming the body and inducing a state of rest, digestion and repair. "It should be bringing down stress hormones, cooling inflammation, and restoring energy to digestion, reproduction and so on," says Stacie Stephenson, DC, who's based in the Chicago area. Stephenson serves as chair of functional medicine for Cancer Treatment

Centers of America and is the author of *Vibrant: A Groundbreaking Program to Get Energized, Own Your Health, and Glow.* "But in a state of chronic stress, the sympathetic nervous system stays in control, inflammation becomes systemic, digestion becomes disrupted, fertility may go offline, and you're in a state of perpetual stress without that all-important recovery."

A study published in *Frontiers in Human Neuroscience* calls chronic, low-grade inflammation "the common soil" of stress-related diseases. "Stressful events engender multiple neurochemical, neurotransmitter and hormonal alterations by mainly activating the sympathetic nervous system (SNS) and the hypothalamic-pituitary-adrenal (HPA) axis," the study reports. "Stress is the common risk factor of 75% to 90% of diseases, including the diseases which cause the foremost morbidity and mortality." These include cardiovascular diseases, diabetes, cancer, depression, Alzheimer's and Parkinson's.

One Coin, Two Sides

All stress is not the same, though. Beneficial stress, also called eustress, improves your health by creating resiliency. Good physical stress, for example, would include exercise, spending time in an infrared sauna, cryotherapy and intermittent fasting—these push the body a bit, triggering a positive response, such as building muscle, increasing blood flow and reducing inflammation. The source of the stress matters too: The kind you have forced upon you, such as the loss of a loved one, tends to be more negative than chosen stress, like going back to pursue a graduate degree. But regardless of the cause, stress becomes negative when there's so much of it, the body can't return to homeostasis, or its internal equilibrium, weakening the body's immune response and capacity for tissue repair.

How do you know if stress is causing inflammation? Watch out for vague, unexplained symptoms such as joint pain, digestive troubles, frequent headaches, feeling fatigued or insomnia. The best way to test for inflammation, Stephenson says, is to get a high-sensitivity C-reactive protein test, or hs-CRP. "This is sometimes called a cardiac CRP test because it is a good measure of acute inflammation that is a risk factor for heart disease," she says. "Another inflammation test is an erythrocyte sedimentation rate or ESR test, which is a more indirect and less sensitive measure of inflammation. If you're not at risk of inflammation but want to know if you have it, your doctor may order an ESR test first. If you have any heart disease risk, however, I suggest requesting the hs-CRP test instead."

Hit the Reset Button

Try these strategies to make stress more manageable.
Enjoy Some Fresh Air According to a study published in the journal *Environmental Research*, exposure to green spaces

> You can order your own blood work at letsgetchecked.com or directlabs.com.

such as parks, woodlands and beaches significantly reduces people's levels of salivary cortisol, used as a marker of stress. Aim to spend at least 120 minutes in nature each week (do that while exercising and you get a stress-relieving "two-fer").
Tune In New types of wearable technology can help retrain the nervous system. Apollo Neuro is a device worn on the ankle or wrist and vibrates to stimulate the parasympathetic nervous system. Muse 2 is a headband that provides feedback on heart rate and other body activity during meditation.
Work Up a Sweat Physical activity reduces levels of stress hormones such as adrenaline and cortisol, and boosts the production of

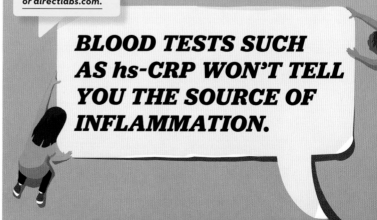

BLOOD TESTS SUCH AS hs-CRP WON'T TELL YOU THE SOURCE OF INFLAMMATION.

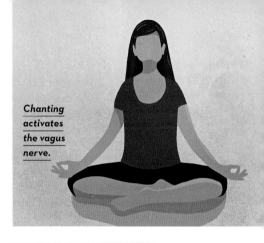

Chanting activates the vagus nerve.

endorphins, elevating the mood. Aim for at least 150 minutes a week. The type of exercise isn't important so much as moving the body regularly. "But give yourself recovery time," says Stephenson. Overtraining triggers negative stress and thwarts benefits.

Tone the Vagus Nerve
The vagus nerve is key in modulating anti-inflammatory and immune system responses. Increasing vagal tone means your body is able to return to the rest/digest phase with more ease, while poor vagal tone means you're having a hard time bouncing back; you're getting stuck in fight-or-flight. "You want to be able to quickly tend to a threat, then return to a calm state," says Owen.

You can "tone" the vagus nerve, which runs through the back of the throat (in the neck), with singing, humming or a quick blast of cold water on your face. You can also do it in the shower by alternating 30 seconds of cold water on your body with 30 seconds of hot water.

Eat (and Supplement) Right
Stephenson suggests downing lots of vegetables, fruit, fiber and omega-3–rich fatty fish. Gamma-aminobutyric acid, or GABA, supplements may protect against stress and anxiety by acting on the nervous system through the gut-brain axis.

Get Connected "Foster healthy relationships for support," says Stephenson—including yourself. "Protect yourself. Love yourself. Take care of yourself, and your immune system will take care of you."

How Trauma Triggers Inflammation

Physical trauma, such as a broken bone, triggers inflammation by both activating immune cells in the area of injury as well as marshaling a systemic inflammatory response. Emotional trauma can do the same, and new research is showing the profound impact that trauma has on children—even decades later. Plus, children who grow up in a chronically stressful state may never learn how to properly calm down their nervous systems. "Our nervous system responds when we perceive threats, and if we do not feel safe, it will not reset to that parasympathetic state," says Leah Owen, MC, LAC.

Childhood trauma—emotional, physical, mental or sexual—is associated with inflammation later in life, measured via markers in the blood such as C-reactive protein (CRP) and the cytokine interleukin-6 (IL-6). That may explain the higher rates of chronic diseases such as arthritis, heart disease and cancer among people who have a history of childhood trauma. Trauma can also be carried from one generation to another. "Children of Holocaust survivors, for example, have higher rates of depression, anxiety and even PTSD," says Owen. "Sometimes, it's a question of, 'How is my body responding to my ancestors' trauma?'"

If you have a history of personal or family trauma, there is hope. The brain and nervous system can be coached on how to reach a restful state, through breath work, meditation practice or other coping skills. Cognitive behavioral therapy (CBT) may also help.

20 Ways to Turn It *Down*

These quick tips will lower the flame, balance your immune system and keep you feeling your best.

1 LOSE EXCESS POUNDS WHITE ADIPOSE TISSUE—WHICH STORES ENERGY BUT ALSO PLAYS A ROLE IN HORMONE REGULATION, HUNGER SIGNALING, INSULIN RELEASE AND IMMUNE SYSTEM CONTROL—CAUSES MORE MACROPHAGES (AN IMMUNE CELL) TO BE RELEASED, WHICH CAN PROMPT MORE INFLAMMATION.

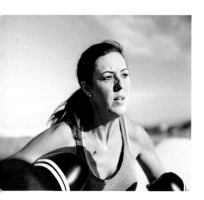

2 *TAKE A REST* Too much intense cardio in a week or back-to-back-to-back weight sessions can lead to overtraining, which creates stress and triggers inflammation. To give your body time to recover, aim for no more than two or three high-intensity workouts a week and allow your muscles at least 48 hours of rest between workout sessions.

3 *SING A TUNE* The vagus nerve is the main part of the parasympathetic nervous system and is key in modulating anti-inflammatory and immune system responses. Increasing vagal tone, by singing, humming and even taking a cold shower, means your body can return to the rest/digest phase with more ease.

4 *CHECK YOUR PILLS* Over-relying on NSAIDs (ibuprofen and naproxen, in particular) for pain, headaches or other problems can create inflammation by contributing to gut permeability.

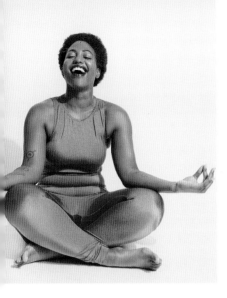

5 GET BENDY RESEARCH HAS SHOWN THAT HATHA YOGA, WHICH INCLUDES YOGA POSES, PRANAYAMA (BREATHING EXERCISES) AND MEDITATION, IMPROVED STRESS AND INFLAMMATORY RESPONSES, BASED ON CHANGES IN CORTISOL, IL-6 (A CYTOKINE THAT MODULATES IMMUNE RESPONSE) AND OTHER FACTORS.

6 PUMP IT UP
Strength training has been shown to help slow the natural decline of immune system function that happens with age and helps keep cognitive function robust. Plus, it preserves muscle and strength as the years tick by, reducing the odds of falling and breaking a bone—or hitting your head.

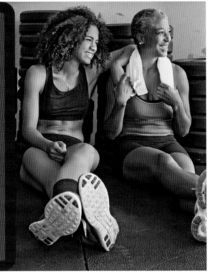

7 INHALE, THEN EXHALE
Rhythmic breathing shifts your brain and body out of fight-or-flight mode, which calms inflammatory responses. Try a 4-7-8 pattern: Inhale for a count of four, hold the breath for seven seconds, then exhale over eight counts. Use this approach when you can't sleep, during meditation practice or anytime you need to hit reset.

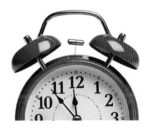

8 KEEP IT CLEAN
Read labels and try to nix foods that contain chemical preservatives and other compounds that may be detrimental to your gut health.

9 SNOOZE MORE GETTING YOUR Z's IS A HUGE PART OF KEEPING YOUR BODY, IMMUNE SYSTEM INCLUDED, WORKING OPTIMALLY. FIND THE SCHEDULE AND HABITS THAT WORK BEST FOR YOU. IF YOU HAVE CHRONIC INSOMNIA, SEE A SLEEP PHYSICIAN.

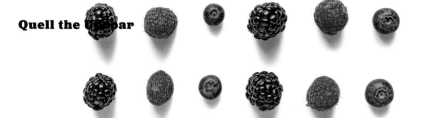

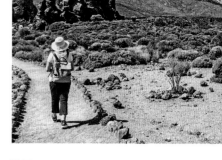

10 BOOST YOUR FIBER

YOU SHOULD DOWN APPROXIMATELY 14 GRAMS OF FIBER FOR EVERY 1,000 CALORIES YOU EAT A DAY, WHICH COMES OUT TO ABOUT 25 GRAMS FOR A WOMAN AND 38 GRAMS FOR A MAN. FIBER KEEPS GOOD BACTERIA HAPPY AND HELPS IMPROVE GUT HEALTH, ENSURING YOU'RE SENDING HEALTHY SIGNALS TO THE REST OF THE BODY.

11 TAKE A HIKE
Spending time in nature helps calm the nervous system. Some research has shown that even looking at pictures of nature will do the trick.

12 STICK TO A ROUTINE
Your body—and innate circadian rhythms— function best on a regular schedule. That means going to bed and getting up at the same time daily and eating at regular times. Throwing this off can trigger inflammation.

13 ROTATE YOUR VEGGIES
Eating the rainbow—a variety of fruits and vegetables of different colors—helps ensure that you get all sorts of healthy plant compounds, including antioxidants, that help squelch inflammation. But let's be clear: Even white veggies such as mushrooms, cauliflower and onions are beneficial, so don't be a veggie colorist.

14 SEE YOUR DENTIST

GUM DISEASE AND SYSTEMIC INFLAMMATION ARE CLOSELY CONNECTED; ONE CAN PROMPT THE OTHER. BRUSH AND FLOSS DAILY AND KEEP UP WITH REGULAR CHECKUPS.

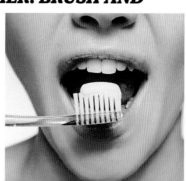

15 SHRINK YOUR WAIST
Even if you don't take off a ton of weight, reducing the size of your belly can help. That's because deep visceral fat that accumulates around (and inside) your organs is more dangerous and inflammatory than the subcutaneous kind. Women should aim for a waist circumference below 35 inches and men below 40 inches.

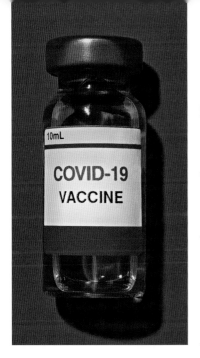

16 *GET VACCINATED!*
THE COVID VACCINE IS SAFE, EFFECTIVE AND FREE. STUDIES HAVE SHOWN IT CAN BOTH REDUCE YOUR RISK OF GETTING THE VIRUS, INCLUDING MANY VARIANTS, AND THE SEVERITY OF SYMPTOMS IF YOU DO CATCH IT. ONE OF THE REASONS THE VIRUS CAN BE SO DANGEROUS IS THE OUTSIZE INFLAMMATORY RESPONSE IT CAN CAUSE.

17 BUTT OUT
Quit smoking, vaping and chewing. There's zero benefit to this habit and it will only harm your health. All those toxic chemicals in tobacco are wreaking havoc in your body.

18 BUST A MOVE
Crime, pollution and toxins in your home or surrounding neighborhood set you up for inflammation and a number of health conditions, including heart disease, depression, asthma and obesity. If you can swing a move financially—and safely—get out.

19 DO A LITTLE SLEUTHING
Feeling bloated, achy, gassy or just unwell? Check your diet to see if certain foods, including dairy, soy, seafood, tree nuts, sugar or gluten are making you feel worse. It's easy to do an elimination diet and sometimes a simple (but not pleasant) program such as Whole30 will show you how good you can feel when you get some of the junk out of your diet.

20 ADD SOME SPICE
Bringing the zing, heat or fire to your food with herbs and spices, including turmeric, cayenne, ginger and garlic, adds not just flavor but anti-inflammatory compounds.

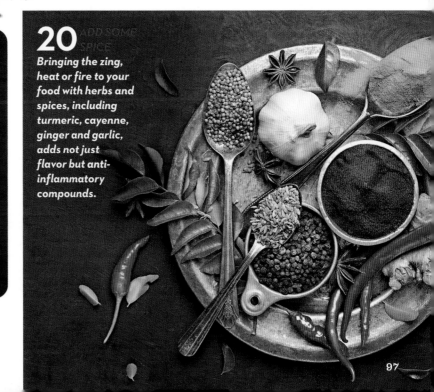

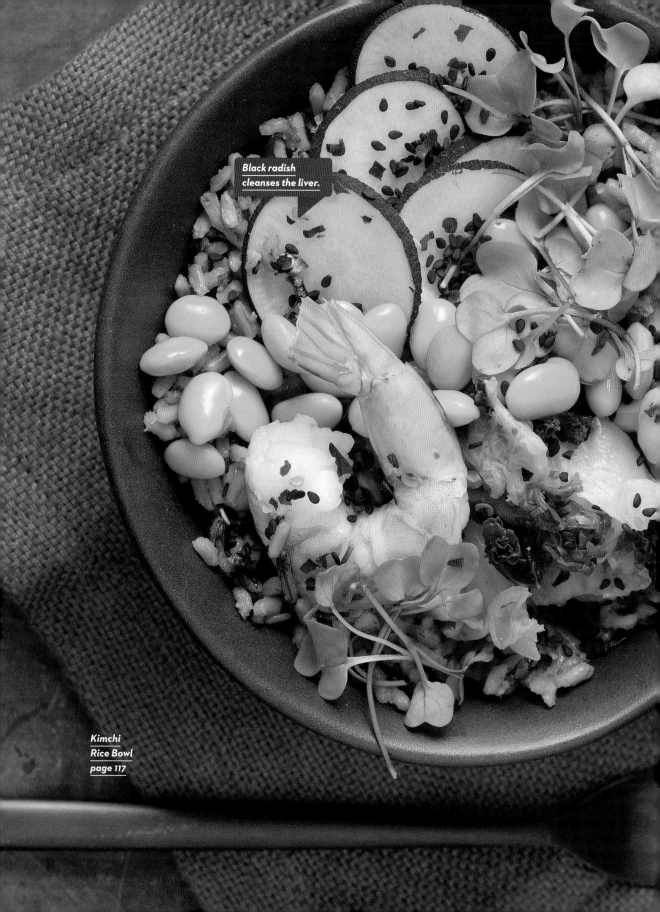

Black radish cleanses the liver.

*Kimchi
Rice Bowl*
page 117

Soothing Recipes

Find 53 meal ideas to fight inflammation,
including satisfying breakfast, lunch,
dinner and dessert options.

MICROGREENS ADD COLOR AND NUTRIENTS.

Asparagus and Avocado Toast With Hard-Boiled Eggs

Avocados are packed with potassium, magnesium, fiber and healthy fats. Research shows they may also help reduce inflammation throughout the body.

PREP 5 minutes
TOTAL 15 minutes
SERVINGS 4

INGREDIENTS

- 2 avocados, halved and pitted
- 1 teaspoon sea salt
- 1 teaspoon lime juice
- 4 slices crusty sourdough bread, toasted
- 20 thin asparagus spears, trimmed and steamed
- 4 hard-boiled eggs, sliced
- 2 teaspoons Aleppo pepper
- 4 tablespoons microgreens or watercress

INSTRUCTIONS

1 In a small bowl, mash avocado with salt and lime juice.
2 Spread mixture evenly over the 4 toast pieces.
3 Top each toast with 5 asparagus spears and then with sliced eggs.
4 Sprinkle evenly with Aleppo pepper and microgreens to serve.

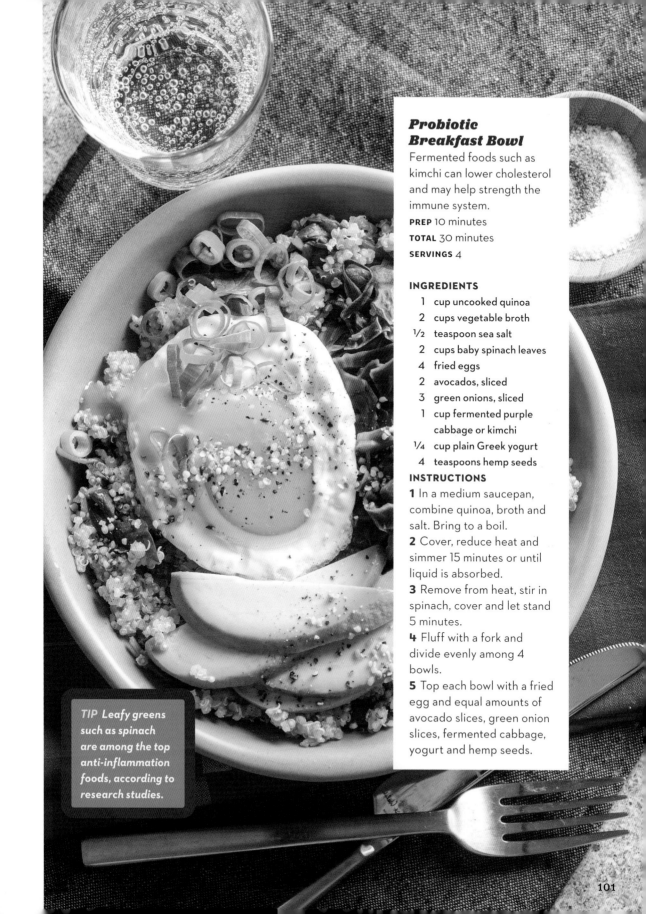

Probiotic Breakfast Bowl

Fermented foods such as kimchi can lower cholesterol and may help strength the immune system.

PREP 10 minutes
TOTAL 30 minutes
SERVINGS 4

INGREDIENTS
- 1 cup uncooked quinoa
- 2 cups vegetable broth
- 1/2 teaspoon sea salt
- 2 cups baby spinach leaves
- 4 fried eggs
- 2 avocados, sliced
- 3 green onions, sliced
- 1 cup fermented purple cabbage or kimchi
- 1/4 cup plain Greek yogurt
- 4 teaspoons hemp seeds

INSTRUCTIONS
1 In a medium saucepan, combine quinoa, broth and salt. Bring to a boil.
2 Cover, reduce heat and simmer 15 minutes or until liquid is absorbed.
3 Remove from heat, stir in spinach, cover and let stand 5 minutes.
4 Fluff with a fork and divide evenly among 4 bowls.
5 Top each bowl with a fried egg and equal amounts of avocado slices, green onion slices, fermented cabbage, yogurt and hemp seeds.

TIP Leafy greens such as spinach are among the top anti-inflammation foods, according to research studies.

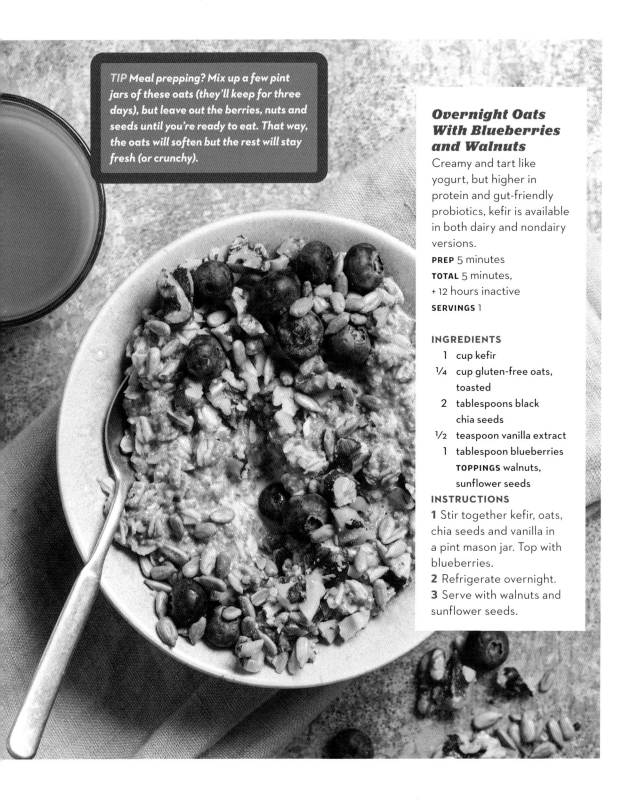

TIP *Meal prepping? Mix up a few pint jars of these oats (they'll keep for three days), but leave out the berries, nuts and seeds until you're ready to eat. That way, the oats will soften but the rest will stay fresh (or crunchy).*

Overnight Oats With Blueberries and Walnuts

Creamy and tart like yogurt, but higher in protein and gut-friendly probiotics, kefir is available in both dairy and nondairy versions.

PREP 5 minutes
TOTAL 5 minutes, + 12 hours inactive
SERVINGS 1

INGREDIENTS
- 1 cup kefir
- ¼ cup gluten-free oats, toasted
- 2 tablespoons black chia seeds
- ½ teaspoon vanilla extract
- 1 tablespoon blueberries
- **TOPPINGS** walnuts, sunflower seeds

INSTRUCTIONS
1 Stir together kefir, oats, chia seeds and vanilla in a pint mason jar. Top with blueberries.
2 Refrigerate overnight.
3 Serve with walnuts and sunflower seeds.

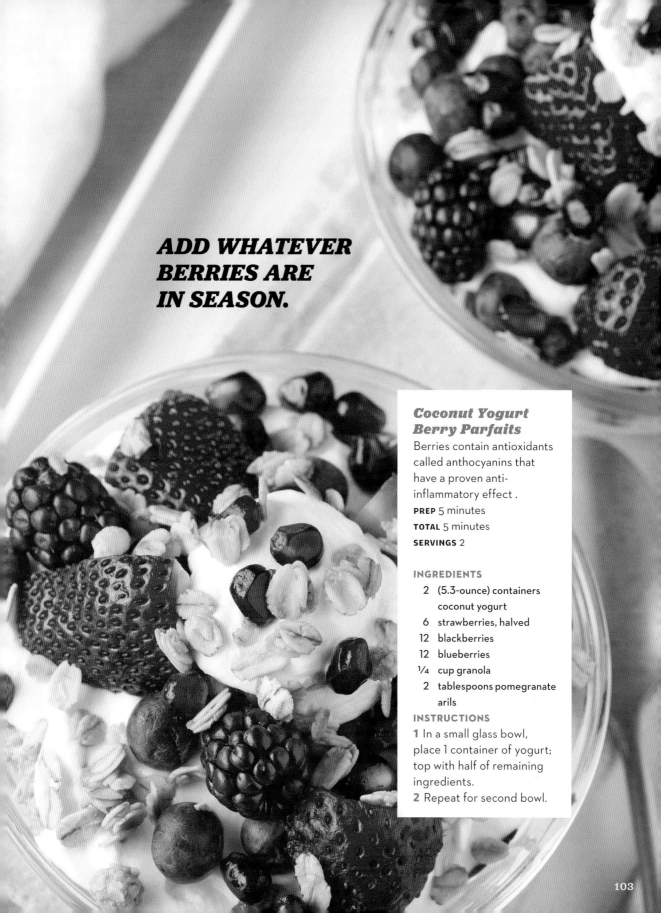

ADD WHATEVER BERRIES ARE IN SEASON.

Coconut Yogurt Berry Parfaits

Berries contain antioxidants called anthocyanins that have a proven anti-inflammatory effect .

PREP 5 minutes
TOTAL 5 minutes
SERVINGS 2

INGREDIENTS

- 2 (5.3-ounce) containers coconut yogurt
- 6 strawberries, halved
- 12 blackberries
- 12 blueberries
- ¼ cup granola
- 2 tablespoons pomegranate arils

INSTRUCTIONS

1 In a small glass bowl, place 1 container of yogurt; top with half of remaining ingredients.

2 Repeat for second bowl.

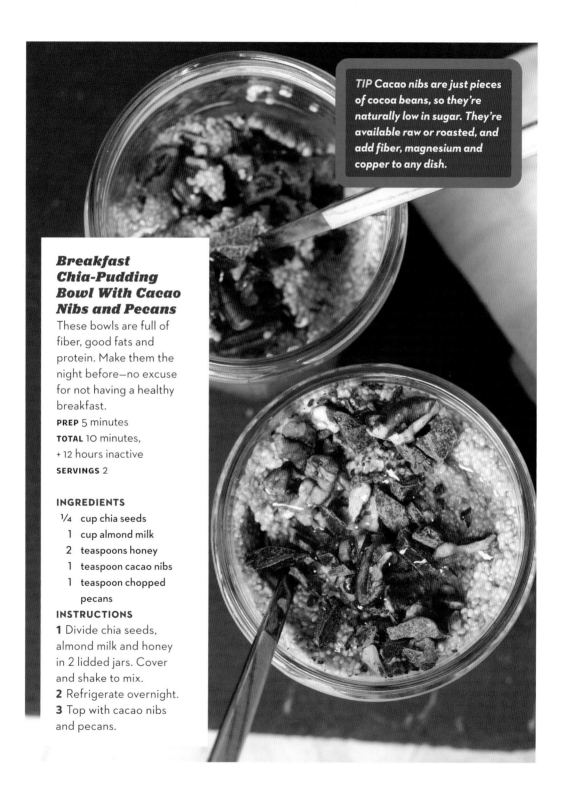

TIP *Cacao nibs are just pieces of cocoa beans, so they're naturally low in sugar. They're available raw or roasted, and add fiber, magnesium and copper to any dish.*

Breakfast Chia-Pudding Bowl With Cacao Nibs and Pecans

These bowls are full of fiber, good fats and protein. Make them the night before—no excuse for not having a healthy breakfast.

PREP 5 minutes

TOTAL 10 minutes, + 12 hours inactive

SERVINGS 2

INGREDIENTS

- ¼ cup chia seeds
- 1 cup almond milk
- 2 teaspoons honey
- 1 teaspoon cacao nibs
- 1 teaspoon chopped pecans

INSTRUCTIONS

1 Divide chia seeds, almond milk and honey in 2 lidded jars. Cover and shake to mix.
2 Refrigerate overnight.
3 Top with cacao nibs and pecans.

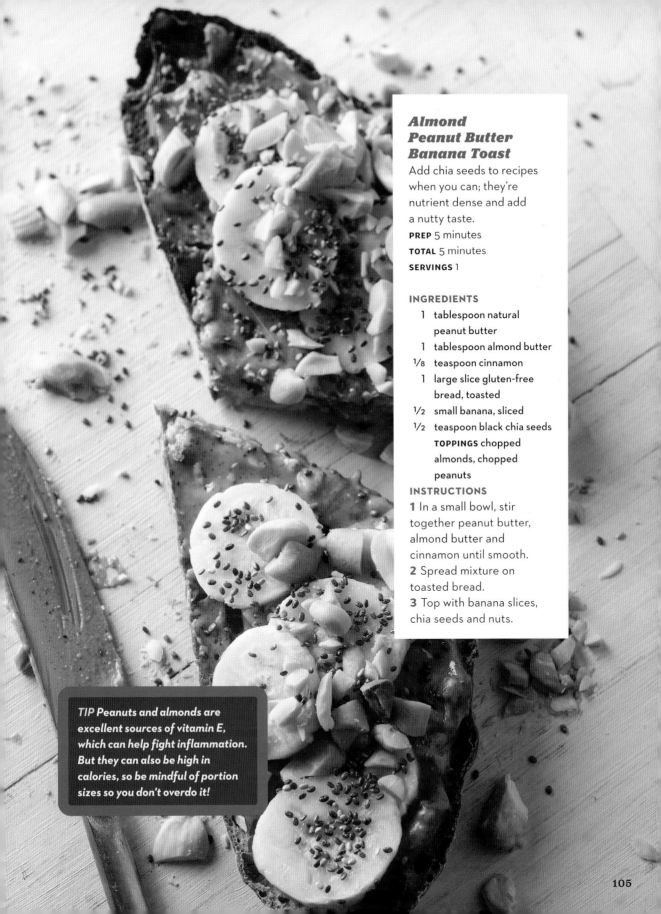

Almond Peanut Butter Banana Toast

Add chia seeds to recipes when you can; they're nutrient dense and add a nutty taste.

PREP 5 minutes
TOTAL 5 minutes
SERVINGS 1

INGREDIENTS

- 1 tablespoon natural peanut butter
- 1 tablespoon almond butter
- 1/8 teaspoon cinnamon
- 1 large slice gluten-free bread, toasted
- 1/2 small banana, sliced
- 1/2 teaspoon black chia seeds
- **TOPPINGS** chopped almonds, chopped peanuts

INSTRUCTIONS

1 In a small bowl, stir together peanut butter, almond butter and cinnamon until smooth.
2 Spread mixture on toasted bread.
3 Top with banana slices, chia seeds and nuts.

TIP Peanuts and almonds are excellent sources of vitamin E, which can help fight inflammation. But they can also be high in calories, so be mindful of portion sizes so you don't overdo it!

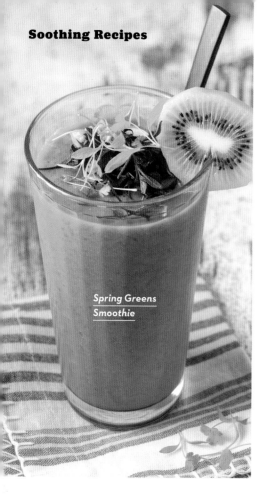

Spring Greens
Smoothie

Cherry Berry Smoothie

Most grocers carry a great variety of frozen berries year-round.

PREP 5 minutes
TOTAL 5 minutes
SERVINGS 2

INGREDIENTS

- 1/2 cup frozen cherries
- 1/2 cup frozen mixed berries
- 1/2 cup almond milk
- 1/2 cup ice cubes
- 1 tablespoon honey
  GARNISH maraschino cherries

INSTRUCTIONS

1 In a blender, mix all ingredients except garnish until smooth.

2 Pour into glasses; garnish as desired.

Spring Greens Smoothie

Kale packs this smoothie full of fiber, antioxidants, calcium and vitamin K—but the mango keeps it all delightfully sweet, while also aiding with the breakdown and digestion of protein.

PREP 5 minutes
TOTAL 5 minutes
SERVINGS 2

INGREDIENTS

- 2 cups kale
- 2 cups spinach
- 2 cups frozen mango chunks
- 2 cups organic, unsweetened apple juice
  GARNISHES kiwi slice, microgreens

INSTRUCTIONS

1 In a blender, mix all ingredients except garnishes until smooth. Pour into glasses.
2 Garnish as desired.

Tropical Smoothie Bowl

Many smoothies start with frozen banana slices. To ensure you always have some on hand, slice up a bunch, put portions in zip-close bags and stash in the freezer.

PREP 5 minutes
TOTAL 5 minutes
SERVINGS 2

INGREDIENTS

- 2 bananas, sliced and frozen
- 2 cups frozen mango pieces
- 2 cups frozen pineapple pieces
- 2 cups coconut milk
  GARNISHES star fruit, chopped macadamia nuts, toasted coconut flakes, black chia seeds, orchid blossoms

INSTRUCTIONS

1 In a blender, mix all ingredients except garnishes until smooth.
2 Pour into bowls; garnish as desired.

Flax-Mocha Smoothie

Flaxseed is an easy way to add inflammation-fighting omega-3s to your diet. Caffeine sensitive? Make this with decaf.

PREP 5 minutes
TOTAL 5 minutes
SERVINGS 2

INGREDIENTS

- 2 cup ice cubes
- 1 1/2 cups plain Greek yogurt
- 1/2 cup cold-brew coffee
- 4 tablespoons ground flaxseed
- 1 tablespoon unsweetened cocoa
- 4 teaspoons honey
- 1 teaspoon vanilla
  GARNISHES cocoa powder, mint sprig

INSTRUCTIONS

1 In a blender, mix all ingredients except garnishes until smooth.
2 Pour into glasses; garnish as desired.

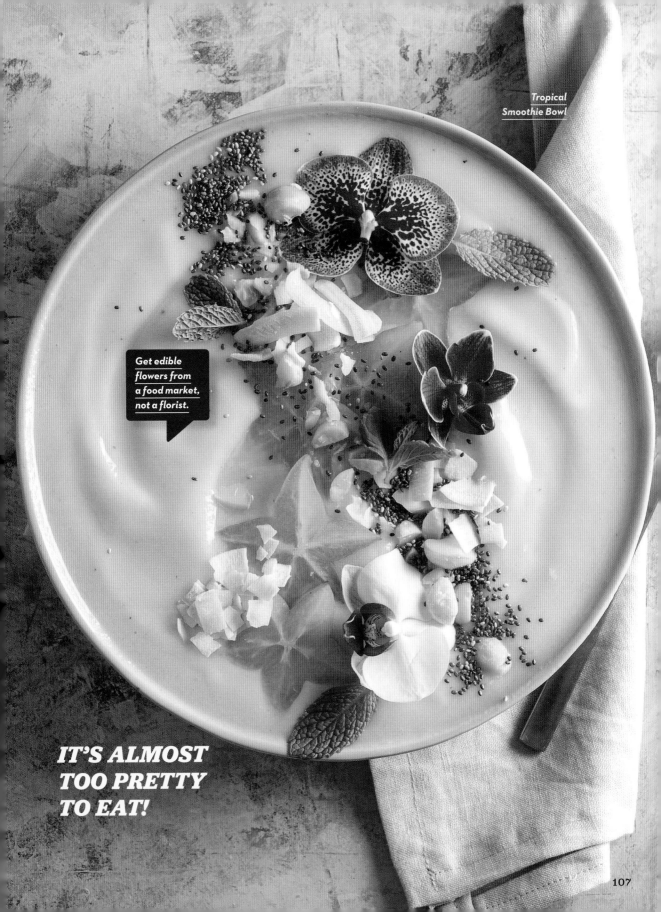

Tropical
Smoothie Bowl

Get edible
flowers from
a food market,
not a florist.

IT'S ALMOST
TOO PRETTY
TO EAT!

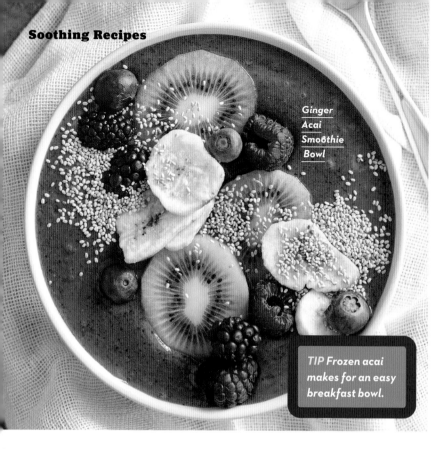

Ginger Acai Smoothie Bowl

TIP *Frozen acai makes for an easy breakfast bowl.*

1 tablespoon flaxseed
1 tablespoon honey or agave syrup

INSTRUCTIONS

1 In a blender, combine all ingredients and blend until smooth.
2 Pour into 2 glasses and serve immediately.

Ginger Acai Smoothie Bowl

This bowl features the superfood acai, which you can find in the frozen section of most supermarkets. Ginger is another powerful food shown to help reduce inflammation.

PREP 5 minutes
TOTAL 5 minutes
SERVINGS 2

INGREDIENTS

2 bananas, sliced and frozen
2 cups frozen mixed berries
1 cup plain Greek yogurt
1 cup almond milk
2 (2-ounce) packets frozen unsweetened acai puree
2 teaspoons minced fresh ginger
  GARNISHES sliced banana chips, blackberries, sliced kiwi, raspberries, blueberries, white chia seeds

Dark Chocolate Avocado Smoothie

Avocado adds plenty of nutrition benefits and creaminess.

PREP 5 minutes
TOTAL 5 minutes
SERVINGS 2

INGREDIENTS

1 ripe avocado, peeled, pitted and cut into chunks
1½ cups unsweetened almond milk
3 tablespoons dark cocoa powder
3 tablespoons honey
2 teaspoons vanilla extract
10 ice cubes

INSTRUCTIONS

1 In a blender, combine all ingredients except ice and blend until smooth.

2 Add ice cubes; process until thick and creamy. Pour into 2 glasses; serve immediately.

Banana-Peach Smoothie

Bright and tangy peaches are packed with antioxidants. Frozen fruits keep your smoothies thick.

PREP 5 minutes
TOTAL 5 minutes
SERVINGS 2

INGREDIENTS

1 cup frozen mango chunks
1 cup frozen sliced peaches
¼ cup peach nectar
1 (6-ounce) container plain Greek yogurt
1 banana, sliced and frozen
¼ cup almond milk

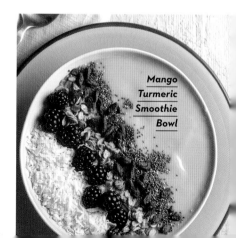

Mango Turmeric Smoothie Bowl

INSTRUCTIONS

1 In a blender, mix all ingredients except garnishes until smooth.

2 Pour into bowls; garnish as desired.

Mango Turmeric Smoothie Bowl

Turmeric is known for its anti-inflammatory powers; goji berries provide immunity-boosting vitamins A,C and E.

PREP 5 minutes

TOTAL 5 minutes

SERVINGS 2

INGREDIENTS

- 4 cups frozen mango chunks
- 2 large bananas, peeled
- 1 cup almond milk
- 2 tablespoons lime juice
- ½ teaspoon turmeric
  GARNISHES blackberries, goji berries, granola, black chia seeds, shredded coconut

INSTRUCTIONS

1 In a blender, combine all ingredients except garnishes and blend until smooth.

2 Pour into bowls; garnish with desired toppings.

Almond Raspberry Smoothie

Almond milk gives a subtle nuttiness to this smoothie. Adjust the amount of agave syrup to your taste.

PREP 5 minutes

TOTAL 5 minutes

SERVINGS 2

INGREDIENTS

- 2 cups frozen raspberries
- 2 cups almond milk
- ⅓ cup almond butter
- ¼ cup agave syrup (optional)
  GARNISHES sliced Marcona almonds, raspberries

INSTRUCTIONS

1 In a blender, combine all ingredients except garnishes. Blend until smooth.

2 Pour into glasses; garnish as desired.

Apricot-Strawberry Smoothie

This simple, three-ingredient smoothie will keep you powered up till lunchtime. Apricots contain antioxidants that are hard to find in other foods. Don't peel them; there's plenty of fiber and nutrients in the skin.

PREP 5 minutes

TOTAL 5 minutes

SERVINGS 2

INGREDIENTS

- 2 cups frozen strawberries
- ½ cup unsweetened cashew or almond milk
- 4 fresh or frozen apricots, pitted and sliced

INSTRUCTIONS

1 In a blender, mix all of the ingredients until they are smooth.

2 Serve immediately; garnish with additional strawberries if desired.

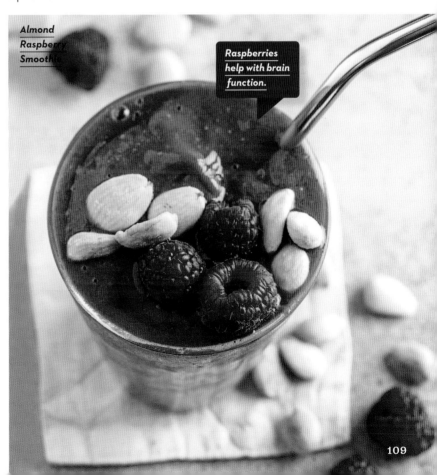

Almond Raspberry Smoothie

Raspberries help with brain function.

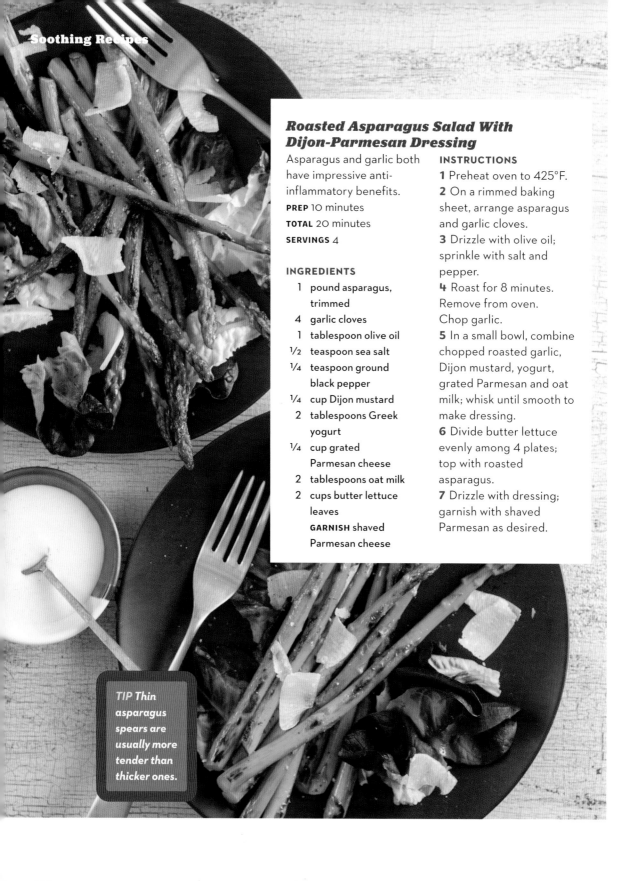

Roasted Asparagus Salad With Dijon-Parmesan Dressing

Asparagus and garlic both have impressive anti-inflammatory benefits.

PREP 10 minutes
TOTAL 20 minutes
SERVINGS 4

INGREDIENTS

- 1 pound asparagus, trimmed
- 4 garlic cloves
- 1 tablespoon olive oil
- ½ teaspoon sea salt
- ¼ teaspoon ground black pepper
- ¼ cup Dijon mustard
- 2 tablespoons Greek yogurt
- ¼ cup grated Parmesan cheese
- 2 tablespoons oat milk
- 2 cups butter lettuce leaves
- **GARNISH** shaved Parmesan cheese

INSTRUCTIONS

1 Preheat oven to 425°F.
2 On a rimmed baking sheet, arrange asparagus and garlic cloves.
3 Drizzle with olive oil; sprinkle with salt and pepper.
4 Roast for 8 minutes. Remove from oven. Chop garlic.
5 In a small bowl, combine chopped roasted garlic, Dijon mustard, yogurt, grated Parmesan and oat milk; whisk until smooth to make dressing.
6 Divide butter lettuce evenly among 4 plates; top with roasted asparagus.
7 Drizzle with dressing; garnish with shaved Parmesan as desired.

TIP Thin asparagus spears are usually more tender than thicker ones.

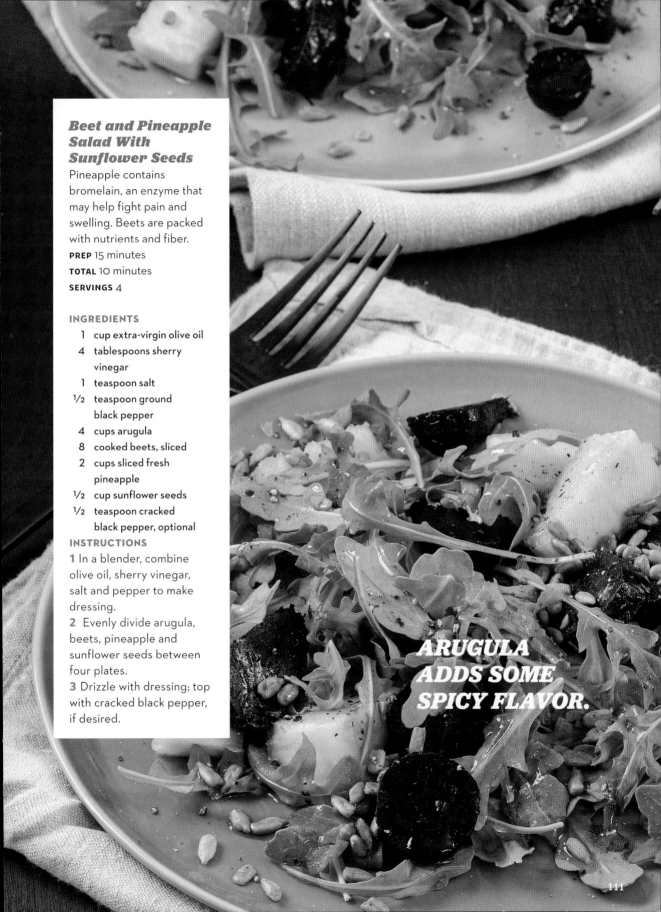

Beet and Pineapple Salad With Sunflower Seeds

Pineapple contains bromelain, an enzyme that may help fight pain and swelling. Beets are packed with nutrients and fiber.

PREP 15 minutes

TOTAL 10 minutes

SERVINGS 4

INGREDIENTS

- 1 cup extra-virgin olive oil
- 4 tablespoons sherry vinegar
- 1 teaspoon salt
- ½ teaspoon ground black pepper
- 4 cups arugula
- 8 cooked beets, sliced
- 2 cups sliced fresh pineapple
- ½ cup sunflower seeds
- ½ teaspoon cracked black pepper, optional

INSTRUCTIONS

1 In a blender, combine olive oil, sherry vinegar, salt and pepper to make dressing.

2 Evenly divide arugula, beets, pineapple and sunflower seeds between four plates.

3 Drizzle with dressing; top with cracked black pepper, if desired.

ARUGULA ADDS SOME SPICY FLAVOR.

111

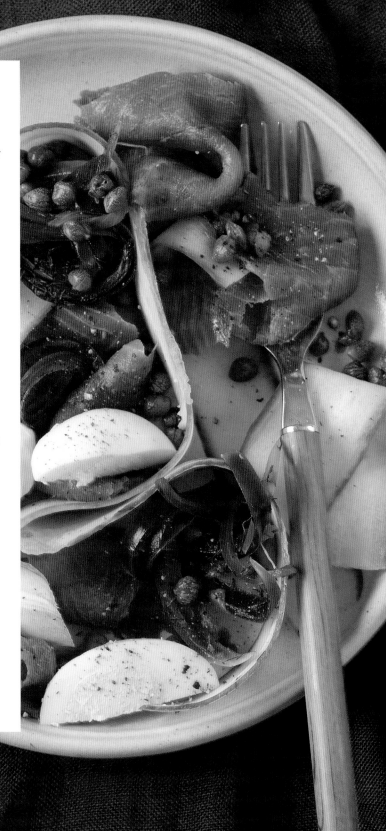

Smoked Salmon Salad With Cucumber Ribbons and Red Onion

Pickled onions and gut-healthy yogurt add a nice tartness to this dish.

PREP 10 minutes

TOTAL 15 minutes
+ 15 minutes inactive

SERVINGS 4

INGREDIENTS

- 1   small red onion, thinly sliced
- 1   cup red wine vinegar
- 1   tablespoon sugar
- ½   teaspoon salt
- 1½ teaspoons dried dill
- 1   (8-ounce) package smoked salmon
- 1   English cucumber, skin on, sliced into ribbons
- 2   hard-boiled eggs, quartered
- ¼   cup Greek yogurt
    Cracked black pepper
    GARNISH capers

INSTRUCTIONS

1 In a small saucepan over medium-high heat, add red onion, vinegar, sugar, salt and dried dill. Bring to a boil. Cover and let stand 15 minutes.

2 On a large platter, arrange salmon pieces, cucumber ribbons, eggs and dollops of yogurt. Drain onion mixture and place on top.

3 Top with cracked pepper and capers and serve.

Shaved Brussels Sprouts Salad With Miso Dressing

Cruciferous vegetables such as Brussels sprouts may reduce the risk of pro-inflammatory diseases. Miso is a traditional Japanese food made from fermented soybeans (and sometimes barley, rice and other ingredients) that is rich in gut-friendly probiotics.

PREP 5 minutes

TOTAL 10 minutes

SERVINGS 4

INGREDIENTS

- ½ cup extra-virgin olive oil
- 3 tablespoons rice wine vinegar
- 1 tablespoon white miso
- ½ teaspoon salt
- ½ teaspoon ground black pepper
- 2 (9-ounce) bags shaved Brussels sprouts
- **GARNISHES** red pepper flakes, lemon wedges

INSTRUCTIONS

1 In a blender, add olive oil, vinegar, miso, salt and pepper; blend until smooth to make dressing.

2 In a large bowl, toss Brussels sprouts with dressing.

3 Garnish as desired and serve.

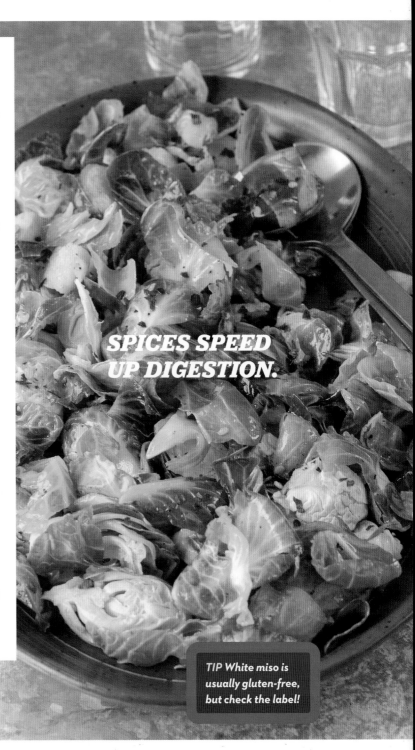

SPICES SPEED UP DIGESTION.

TIP White miso is usually gluten-free, but check the label!

Quinoa Tabbouleh Salad With Tomatoes, Cucumber and Mint

Traditionally, bulgur wheat is used in tabbouleh, but quinoa makes a low-fat, high-protein substitute that's equally tasty.

PREP 10 minutes
TOTAL 30 minutes
SERVINGS 4

INGREDIENTS

- 1   cup quinoa
- 2   cups water
- ¾   teaspoon sea salt, divided
- 1   cup chopped parsley
- ¼   cup coarsely chopped mint
- ½   cup extra-virgin olive oil
- 2   tablespoons lemon juice
- 1   teaspoon chopped garlic
- ¼   teaspoon ground black pepper
- 1   pint grape tomatoes
- 1   English cucumber, sliced in half-moons
- ¼   teaspoon ground black pepper
- **GARNISH** mint leaves

INSTRUCTIONS

1 In a medium saucepan, combine quinoa, water and ½ teaspoon salt.

2 Over medium-high heat, bring to a boil. Reduce heat to medium low; cover and simmer for 15 minutes or until all the water is evaporated.

3 Remove from heat and let stand for 5 minutes. Fluff with a fork. Let cool.

4 Meanwhile, in a small bowl, combine parsley, mint, olive oil, lemon juice, garlic, and remaining sea salt and pepper; mix well to make dressing.

5 In a large bowl, combine cooled quinoa, dressing, tomatoes and cucumber slices.

6 Garnish with black pepper and mint leaves as desired.

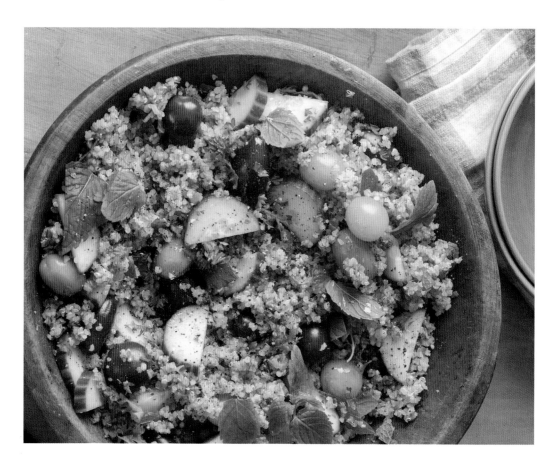

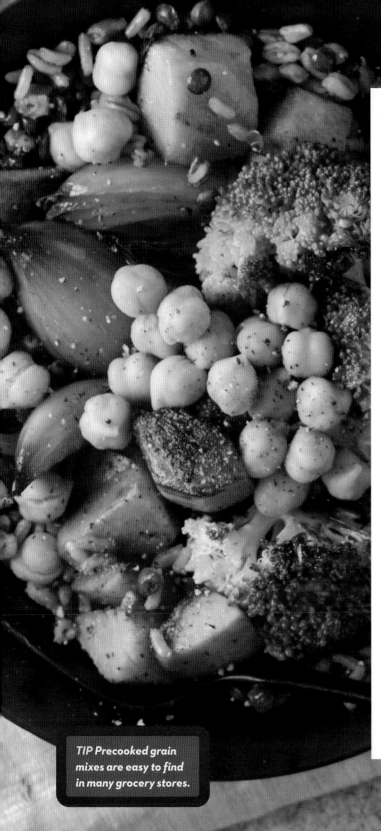

TIP Precooked grain mixes are easy to find in many grocery stores.

Chickpea and Spelt Bowl With Roasted Broccoli and Shallots

Spelt is an ancient grain. It is an excellent source of dietary fiber. It is also rich in iron, magnesium, phosphorus and zinc.

PREP 15 minutes

TOTAL 25 minutes

SERVINGS 2

INGREDIENTS

- 1 cup broccoli florets
- 2 shallots, quartered
- 1 cup cubed butternut squash
- 1 tablespoon avocado or olive oil
- ½ teaspoon sea salt
- ½ teaspoon ground black pepper
- 1 (8-ounce) package microwaveable spelt, green lentils and long-grain brown rice, cooked according to package directions
- 1 (15.5-ounce) can garbanzo beans, drained and rinsed

INSTRUCTIONS

1 Preheat oven to 400°F.

2 On a rimmed sheet pan, place broccoli florets, shallots and squash. Drizzle with oil; sprinkle with salt and pepper.

3 Roast in oven for 10 minutes or until vegetables are browned, flipping halfway through cooking. Remove from oven.

4 Divide the spelt, green lentils and brown rice mix between 2 individual serving bowls.

5 Top each bowl with roasted vegetables and garbanzo beans.

Citrus Chicken Salad Bowl

This colorful meal makes a tasty lunch to pack for the office or school.

PREP 10 minutes
TOTAL 15 minutes
SERVINGS 2

INGREDIENTS

- 1 (8-ounce) bag organic fully cooked coconut rice
- 1 cup cooked chicken breast, sliced
- ½ cup chopped celery
- 1 small orange, sectioned
- 1 cup purple cabbage, thinly sliced
- ½ cup pea sprouts
- 1 tablespoon hot sesame oil
- 1 tablespoon tamari
- ⅛ teaspoon red pepper flakes
- **GARNISHES** lime wedges, red pepper flakes

INSTRUCTIONS

1 Heat coconut rice according to package directions.
2 Divide rice evenly between 2 individual serving bowls.
3 Top each with half of the chicken, celery, orange, cabbage and pea sprouts.
4 In a small bowl, whisk together hot sesame oil, tamari and red pepper flakes.
5 Drizzle mixture over bowls.
6 Garnish with lime wedges and red pepper flakes.

Kimchi Rice Bowl

Edamame is an excellent source of protein and other nutrients, while kimchi helps promote a healthy microbiome and fight inflammation.

PREP 5 minutes
TOTAL 10 minutes
SERVINGS 2

INGREDIENTS
- 1 (8.5-ounce) package precooked brown rice/ wild rice medley microwaved according to package directions
- 1 cup kimchi
- 4 jumbo shrimp, cooked
- ½ cup cooked edamame
- ¼ cup black radish slices
- ¼ cup radish microgreens
- ¼ cup rice wine vinegar
  GARNISHES black sesame seeds, red pepper flakes

INSTRUCTIONS
1 Divide rice evenly between 2 individual serving bowls.
2 Top each bowl with half of kimchi, shrimp, edamame, radish and microgreens.
3 Sprinkle each bowl with rice wine vinegar; top with sesame seeds and red pepper flakes.

Grilled Eggplant With Pine Nuts and Mint

Eggplant is rich in phytonutrients and also loaded with fiber, vitamins, minerals and antioxidants.

PREP 5 minutes
TOTAL 10 minutes
SERVINGS 2

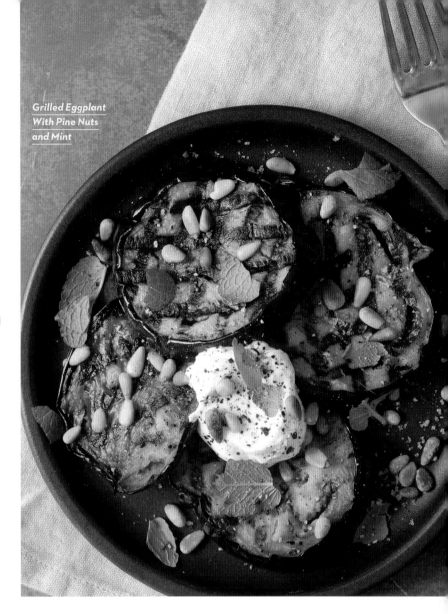

Grilled Eggplant With Pine Nuts and Mint

INGREDIENTS
- 1 small eggplant, cut into thin slices
- 1 tablespoon avocado oil
- ¼ teaspoon salt
- ¼ teaspoon ground black pepper
- 2 tablespoons toasted pine nuts
- ¼ cup plain Greek yogurt
  GARNISH torn mint leaves

INSTRUCTIONS
1 In a medium bowl, toss sliced eggplant with avocado oil, salt and pepper.
2 Place a grill pan over medium-high heat. Place eggplant slices on hot grill; cook 2 minutes per side.
3 Divide eggplant evenly between 2 individual serving bowls.
4 Top each bowl with half of the pine nuts and yogurt. Garnish with mint leaves.

Pumpkin Curry Soup

Not just for Halloween: The vitamin A in pumpkin can strengthen your immune system and help fight infections. Pumpkin is also high in vitamins C and E, iron and folate.

PREP 20 minutes
TOTAL 40 minutes
SERVINGS 4

INGREDIENTS

- 1   tablespoon olive oil
- 1   teaspoon minced garlic
- 2   teaspoons curry powder
- 2   pounds pumpkin, peeled and cubed
- 1   (32-ounce) box vegetable broth
- ¼   teaspoon sea salt
- ¼   teaspoon ground black pepper
- 1   (13.5-ounce) can coconut milk
     GARNISHES cilantro leaves, toasted coconut flakes

INSTRUCTIONS

1 In a Dutch oven over medium-high heat, heat olive oil for 1 minute. Stir in garlic and curry powder.
2 Add pumpkin, broth, salt and pepper and bring to a boil. Reduce heat; simmer for 20 minutes or until pumpkin is tender.
3 Stir in coconut milk. Using an immersion blender, blend until smooth.
4 Garnish as desired to serve.

Turmeric Chicken Zoodle Soup

This warming soup is filled with disease-fighting, vitamin-packed ingredients.

PREP 15 minutes
TOTAL 1 hour
SERVINGS 4

INGREDIENTS

- 2   tablespoons avocado oil
- 1   large onion, chopped
- 1   teaspoon chopped garlic
- ½   cup chopped celery
- 1   cup sliced carrots
- 2   bay leaves
- 1   teaspoon turmeric
- 1   tablespoon apple cider vinegar
- 2   cups chicken bone broth (see recipe, opposite page) or chicken broth
- 1   cup canned pumpkin
- 3   cups chopped kale
- 2   cups shredded rotisserie chicken
- 1   (16-ounce) container zucchini "zoodles' (or make your own with a spiralizer)
     GARNISH chopped parsley

INSTRUCTIONS

1 In a large stock pot over medium-high heat, heat oil.
2 Add onion, garlic, celery and carrots. Cook for 10 minutes.
3 Add bay leaves, turmeric, vinegar, broth, pumpkin, kale and chicken. Cook for about 30 minutes or until vegetables have softened.
4 Stir in zoodles; cook for 5 minutes. Remove bay leaves and discard.
5 Serve in bowls; garnish as desired.

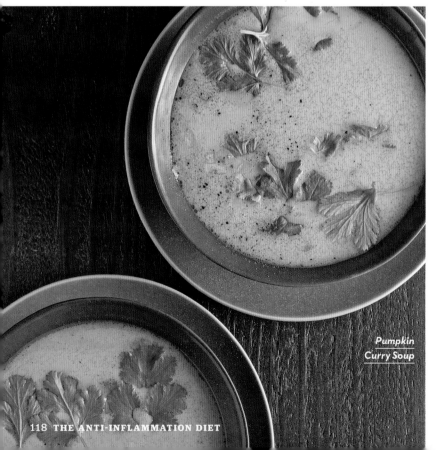

Pumpkin Curry Soup

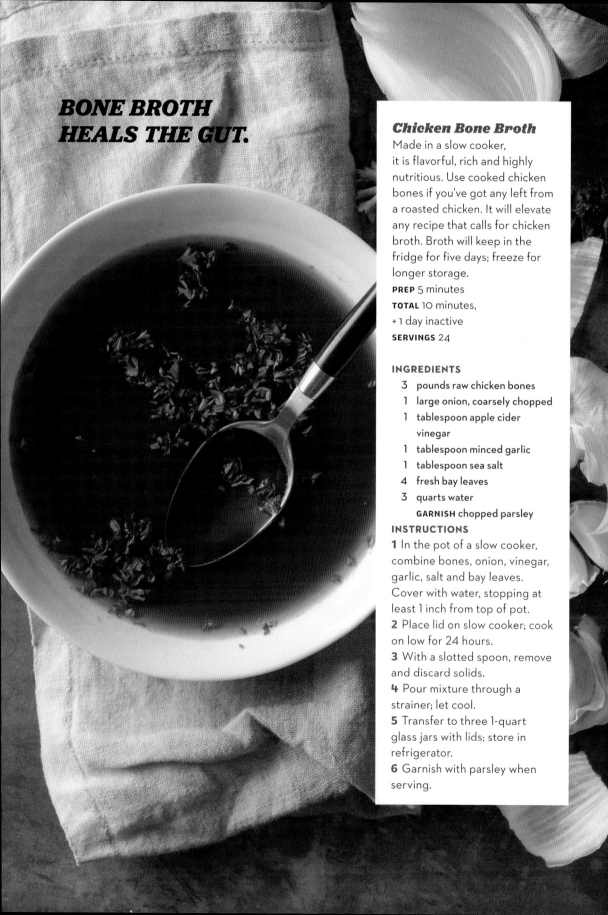

BONE BROTH HEALS THE GUT.

Chicken Bone Broth

Made in a slow cooker, it is flavorful, rich and highly nutritious. Use cooked chicken bones if you've got any left from a roasted chicken. It will elevate any recipe that calls for chicken broth. Broth will keep in the fridge for five days; freeze for longer storage.

PREP 5 minutes
TOTAL 10 minutes, + 1 day inactive
SERVINGS 24

INGREDIENTS

- 3 pounds raw chicken bones
- 1 large onion, coarsely chopped
- 1 tablespoon apple cider vinegar
- 1 tablespoon minced garlic
- 1 tablespoon sea salt
- 4 fresh bay leaves
- 3 quarts water
- **GARNISH** chopped parsley

INSTRUCTIONS

1 In the pot of a slow cooker, combine bones, onion, vinegar, garlic, salt and bay leaves. Cover with water, stopping at least 1 inch from top of pot.
2 Place lid on slow cooker; cook on low for 24 hours.
3 With a slotted spoon, remove and discard solids.
4 Pour mixture through a strainer; let cool.
5 Transfer to three 1-quart glass jars with lids; store in refrigerator.
6 Garnish with parsley when serving.

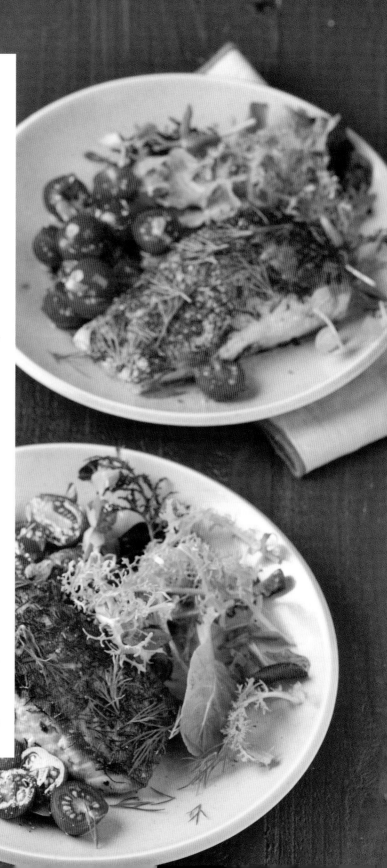

Herb-Crusted Salmon Fillets With Tomato and Oregano Salad

The herbs in this recipe give the salmon a Greek flair. Serve lemon wedges on the side; citrus and fish paired together are a natural combo.

PREP 5 minutes
TOTAL 20 minutes
SERVINGS 4

INGREDIENTS

- 4 (6-ounce) salmon fillets
- ½ teaspoon salt
- ½ teaspoon ground black pepper
- 1 tablespoon chopped chives
- 1 tablespoon dill
- 1 tablespoon thyme
- 2 tablespoons avocado oil
- 1 pint cherry tomatoes, halved
- ¼ cup olive oil
- 2 cups mixed salad greens
  GARNISHES oregano leaves, dill sprigs

INSTRUCTIONS

1 Sprinkle salmon fillets with salt, pepper and herbs.
2 Place avocado oil in a cast iron skillet over medium-high heat.
3 Add fillets to pan and cook 3 minutes per side or until cooked through.
4 Meanwhile, in a large bowl, toss tomato halves with olive oil.
5 Divide salad greens between 4 dinner plates.
6 Top with salmon and tomatoes. Garnish with oregano leaves and dill.

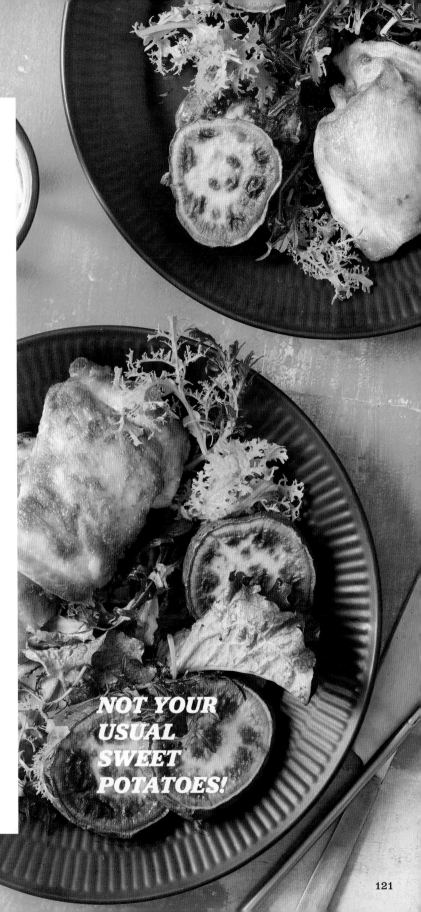

Caribbean Chicken Thighs With Sweet Potatoes and Mixed Greens

The antioxidants and fiber in sweet potatoes are inflammation-fighting warriors.

PREP 5 minutes

TOTAL 25 minutes

SERVINGS 2

INGREDIENTS

- 4 chicken thighs
- 1/2 teaspoon salt
- 1/2 teaspoon ground black pepper
- 2 tablespoons coconut oil, divided
- 1 sweet potato, unpeeled and sliced
- 2 cups organic mixed greens
- 2 tablespoons avocado oil, divided

INSTRUCTIONS

1 Season chicken with salt and pepper.

2 In a cast-iron skillet, heat 1 tablespoon oil over medium-high heat. Add chicken and cook 4 minutes per side, or until cooked through.

3 Remove chicken from skillet; set aside. Add remaining coconut oil.

4 Add sweet potato slices; cook 4 minutes per side.

5 Divide greens between 2 dinner plates; drizzle greens with avocado oil.

6 Serve chicken thighs and sweet potato slices over mixed greens.

NOT YOUR USUAL SWEET POTATOES!

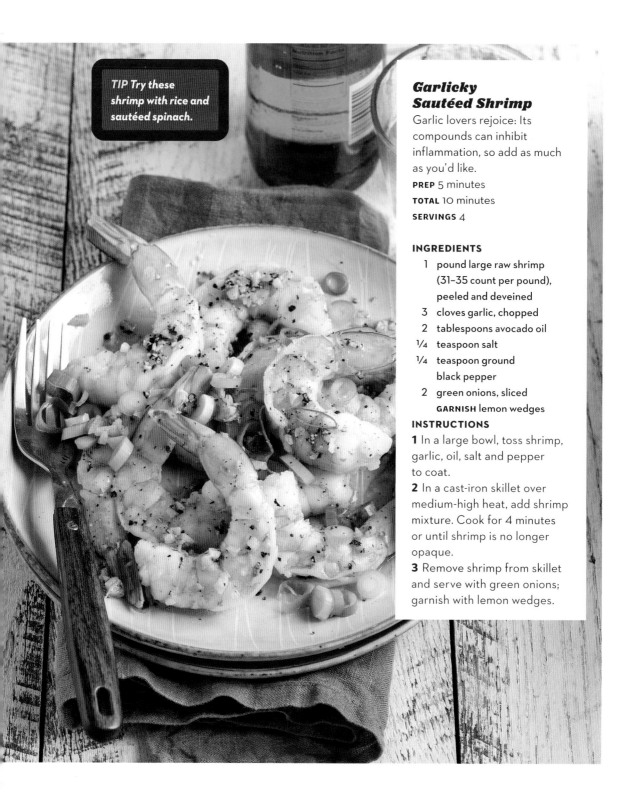

TIP *Try these shrimp with rice and sautéed spinach.*

Garlicky Sautéed Shrimp

Garlic lovers rejoice: Its compounds can inhibit inflammation, so add as much as you'd like.

PREP 5 minutes
TOTAL 10 minutes
SERVINGS 4

INGREDIENTS

- 1 pound large raw shrimp (31–35 count per pound), peeled and deveined
- 3 cloves garlic, chopped
- 2 tablespoons avocado oil
- ¼ teaspoon salt
- ¼ teaspoon ground black pepper
- 2 green onions, sliced
- **GARNISH** lemon wedges

INSTRUCTIONS

1 In a large bowl, toss shrimp, garlic, oil, salt and pepper to coat.

2 In a cast-iron skillet over medium-high heat, add shrimp mixture. Cook for 4 minutes or until shrimp is no longer opaque.

3 Remove shrimp from skillet and serve with green onions; garnish with lemon wedges.

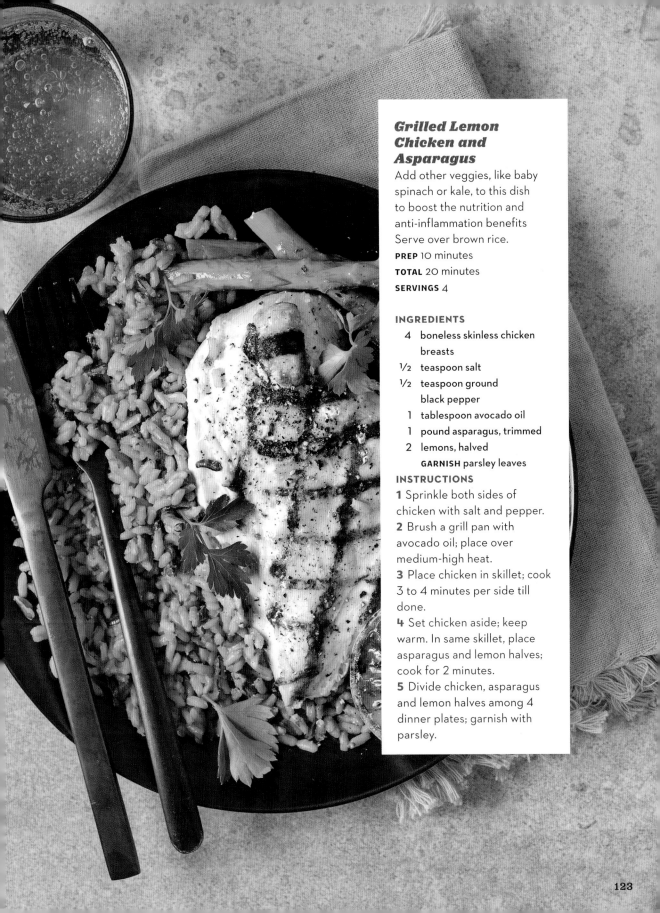

Grilled Lemon Chicken and Asparagus

Add other veggies, like baby spinach or kale, to this dish to boost the nutrition and anti-inflammation benefits Serve over brown rice.

PREP 10 minutes

TOTAL 20 minutes

SERVINGS 4

INGREDIENTS

- 4 boneless skinless chicken breasts
- 1/2 teaspoon salt
- 1/2 teaspoon ground black pepper
- 1 tablespoon avocado oil
- 1 pound asparagus, trimmed
- 2 lemons, halved
- GARNISH parsley leaves

INSTRUCTIONS

1 Sprinkle both sides of chicken with salt and pepper.

2 Brush a grill pan with avocado oil; place over medium-high heat.

3 Place chicken in skillet; cook 3 to 4 minutes per side till done.

4 Set chicken aside; keep warm. In same skillet, place asparagus and lemon halves; cook for 2 minutes.

5 Divide chicken, asparagus and lemon halves among 4 dinner plates; garnish with parsley.

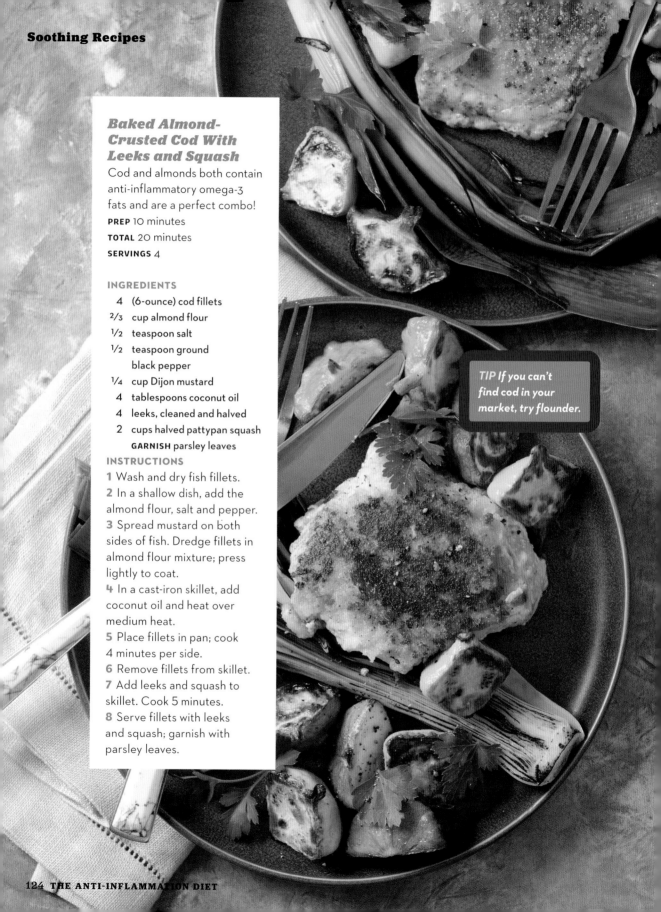

Baked Almond-Crusted Cod With Leeks and Squash

Cod and almonds both contain anti-inflammatory omega-3 fats and are a perfect combo!

PREP 10 minutes
TOTAL 20 minutes
SERVINGS 4

INGREDIENTS

- 4 (6-ounce) cod fillets
- 2/3 cup almond flour
- 1/2 teaspoon salt
- 1/2 teaspoon ground black pepper
- 1/4 cup Dijon mustard
- 4 tablespoons coconut oil
- 4 leeks, cleaned and halved
- 2 cups halved pattypan squash
- GARNISH parsley leaves

INSTRUCTIONS

1 Wash and dry fish fillets.
2 In a shallow dish, add the almond flour, salt and pepper.
3 Spread mustard on both sides of fish. Dredge fillets in almond flour mixture; press lightly to coat.
4 In a cast-iron skillet, add coconut oil and heat over medium heat.
5 Place fillets in pan; cook 4 minutes per side.
6 Remove fillets from skillet.
7 Add leeks and squash to skillet. Cook 5 minutes.
8 Serve fillets with leeks and squash; garnish with parsley leaves.

TIP If you can't find cod in your market, try flounder.

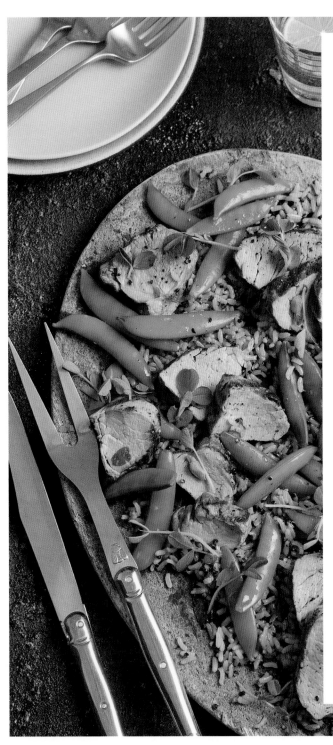

Grilled Pork Tenderloin and Snap Peas

Sugar snap peas are nutritious, satisfying—and totally delicious.

PREP 10 minutes

TOTAL 30 minutes
+ 10 minutes inactive

SERVINGS 4

INGREDIENTS

- 1 pound pork tenderloin
- 1/2 teaspoon granulated garlic
- 1/2 teaspoon salt
- 1/2 teaspoon ground black pepper
- 1 tablespoon olive oil
- 1 (8-ounce) bag sugar snap peas, cooked
- 1 (8.5-ounce) bag red quinoa and brown rice, cooked according to package directions
- GARNISH pea shoots

INSTRUCTIONS

1 Sprinkle all surfaces of pork tenderloin with granulated garlic, salt and pepper.

2 Brush grill pan with olive oil; place over medium-high heat.

3 Grill pork for 18 minutes, turning occasionally, until cooked through.

4 Remove pork from grill; let rest on a cutting board for 10 minutes. Slice into medallions.

5 Divide peas and quinoa mixture evenly between 4 dinner plates; top with pork medallions and garnish with pea shoots as desired.

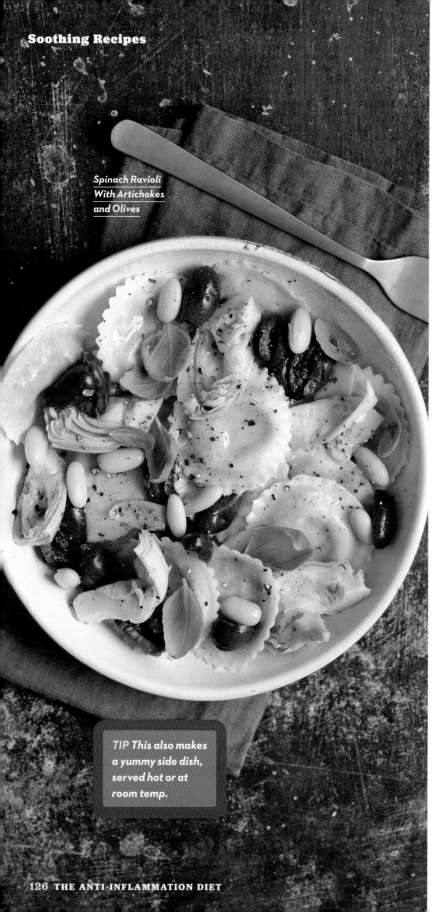

Spinach Ravioli
With Artichokes
and Olives

TIP *This also makes a yummy side dish, served hot or at room temp.*

Spinach Ravioli With Artichokes and Olives

Artichokes are packed with the gut-friendly prebiotic inulin and have more protein than the average veggie, to boot. The jarred hearts are usually marinated in olive oil and lemon or vinegar, so drain them well before using.

PREP 10 minutes
TOTAL 20 minutes
SERVINGS 4

INGREDIENTS

- 1 (8-ounce) package refrigerated spinach-filled ravioli
- ¼ cup olive oil
- ½ teaspoon salt
- ½ teaspoon ground black pepper
- 1 teaspoon chopped garlic
- 1 (12-ounce) jar artichoke hearts, drained
- ½ cup kalamata olives, drained and halved
- 1 (15-ounce) can cannellini beans, drained and rinsed
- **GARNISH** basil leaves

INSTRUCTIONS

1 Cook ravioli according to package directions. Drain; set aside and keep warm.
2 Meanwhile, in a small bowl mix olive oil, salt, pepper and garlic.
3 In a large bowl, combine ravioli, artichoke hearts, olives and beans. Drizzle with olive oil mixture; garnish with basil leaves.

Sesame Garlic Chicken With Broccolini

Broccolini, aka broccoli rabe, is a member of the turnip family; it adds a nutty, earthy, slightly bitter taste and has anti-inflammatory properties.

PREP 5 minutes
TOTAL 15 minutes
SERVINGS 4

INGREDIENTS

- 1 tablespoon sesame oil
- 1 tablespoon chili oil
- 4 boneless, skinless chicken breasts, cubed
- ½ teaspoon salt
- ¼ teaspoon ground black pepper
- 1 (8.8-ounce) package precooked rice, microwaved according to package directions
- 1 (8-ounce) package Broccolini, cooked according to package directions
- ¼ cup cooked edamame
- 1 (12-ounce) bottle garlic-chili sauce
- **GARNISH** red pepper flakes

INSTRUCTIONS

1 In a skillet over medium-high heat, add sesame and chili oils.
2 Sprinkle chicken evenly with salt and pepper. Add chicken to skillet; cook, stirring constantly, for 6 minutes.
3 Meanwhile, divide warm rice evenly among 4 individual serving bowls. Top with cooked chicken, Broccolini and edamame. Drizzle with garlic-chili sauce and garnish with red pepper flakes.

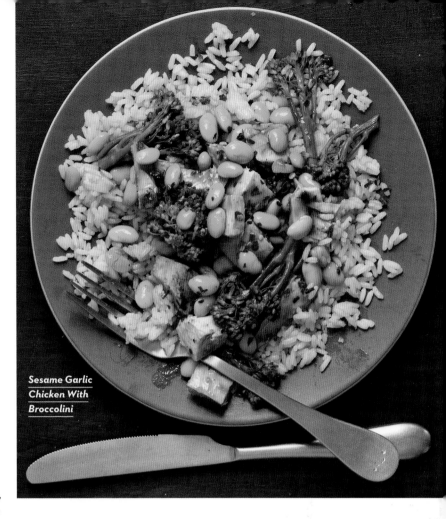

Sesame Garlic Chicken With Broccolini

Butternut Noodles With Parmesan and Herbs

Butternut squash is loaded with antioxidants and makes a great substitute for pasta. Buy the noodles premade to save time or use a spiralizer and make your own. Grate your own Parm cheese for the freshest flavor!

PREP 5 minutes
TOTAL 15 minutes
SERVINGS 4

INGREDIENTS

- ¼ cup ghee
- 6 cups butternut squash noodles
- ½ teaspoon sea salt
- 1 cup grated Parmesan cheese
- ½ teaspoon ground black pepper
- **GARNISHES** torn basil leaves, oregano sprigs

INSTRUCTIONS

1 In a large skillet, melt ghee over medium heat.
2 Add butternut squash noodles and sea salt.
3 Cook until tender, about 8 minutes, tossing occasionally.
4 Remove skillet from heat; stir in Parmesan and pepper.
5 Divide among dinner plates; garnish as desired.

Perfect Bulgur With Savory Toppings

Bulgur is a good source of fiber, which fights inflammation. Try this as a light lunch or as a side for dinner.

PREP 5 minutes
TOTAL 20 minutes
SERVINGS 4

INGREDIENTS

- 4 cups water
- 2 cup bulgur
- 1 teaspoon salt
- ½ teaspoon pepper
- **TOPPINGS** julienned sun-dried tomatoes, basil leaves, fresh corn kernels

INSTRUCTIONS

1 In a saucepan, add water, bulgur, salt and pepper. Bring to a boil.
2 Cover; reduce heat to simmer. Cook for 12 minutes or until water is absorbed.
3 Fluff bulgur with a fork and place in serving bowls.
4 Top with sun-dried tomatoes, basil leaves and corn kernels.

TIP Serve toppings on the side so you can customize your bulgur.

Smoky Baked Chickpeas

Chickpeas are full of protein and soluble fiber, which help increase the number of healthy bacteria in your gut. Double the recipe for a party.

PREP 5 minutes

TOTAL 30 minutes

SERVINGS 4

INGREDIENTS

- 1 (15-ounce) can chickpeas, drained and rinsed
- 1 tablespoon vegetable oil
- 1 teaspoon chili powder
- 1/2 teaspoon cayenne pepper
- 1/2 teaspoon smoked paprika
- 1/2 teaspoon cumin

INSTRUCTIONS

1 Preheat oven to 425°F. Cover a baking sheet with parchment paper.
2 Toss chickpeas with oil and seasonings. Spread on baking sheet.
3 Bake for 25 minutes or until crunchy.
4 Let cool completely.
5 Store in an airtight container for up to 2 weeks.

Kale Chips

Keep a healthy snack like this on hand for those crunch cravings. These are yummy tossed with Parmesan, too. Curly kale works best for this recipe; it holds more seasoning!

PREP 10 minutes

TOTAL 25 minutes

SERVINGS 4

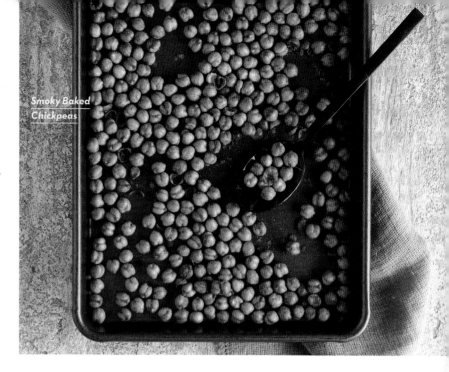

Smoky Baked Chickpeas

INGREDIENTS

- 10 ounces curly kale, trimmed, torn into pieces and well-dried
- 2 tablespoons avocado oil
- 1/2 teaspoon sea salt
- 1/2 teaspoon red pepper flakes

INSTRUCTIONS

1 Preheat oven to 350°F.
2 In a large bowl, toss kale and oil to coat. Sprinkle with salt and pepper and toss again.
3 Place kale in a single layer on a rimmed baking sheet (you may need more than one sheet).
4 Bake for 15 minutes, watching closely to prevent kale from burning.
5 Cool completely. Store in airtight container.

Lemon White Bean Hummus

These beans are high in both protein and fiber, and make a yummy, creamy dip. Serve with crudité or pita chips.

PREP 5 minutes

TOTAL 20 minutes

SERVINGS 4

INGREDIENTS

- 1 (15.5-ounce) can no-salt-added Great Northern beans, drained and rinsed
- 2 tablespoons avocado oil
- 1 tablespoon lemon juice
- 1/2 teaspoon sea salt
- 1/4 teaspoon ground black pepper
- **GARNISH** lemon zest

INSTRUCTIONS

1 In a food processor or blender, mix all ingredients except garnish. Process until smooth, using a spatula to push sides down.
2 Transfer to serving bowl; cover and refrigerate until ready to serve.
3 Garnish with lemon zest right before serving.

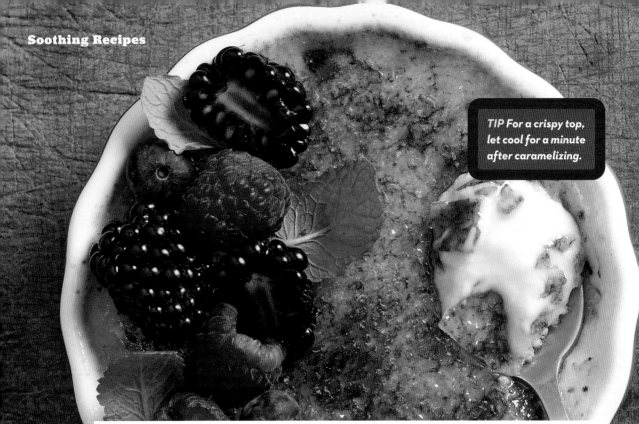

TIP *For a crispy top, let cool for a minute after caramelizing.*

Crème Brûlée With Mixed Berries

This variation on the classic dessert uses coconut milk instead of cream to help fight inflammation.

PREP 15 minutes
TOTAL 1 hour
+ 12 hours inactive
SERVINGS 4

INGREDIENTS

- 2 cups canned coconut milk
- 4 tablespoons honey
- 1 teaspoon salt
- 2 vanilla beans, split and scraped
- 4 egg yolks
- 4 teaspoons maple sugar
- 12 blueberries
- 12 blackberries
- 12 raspberries
- **GARNISH** mint leaves

INSTRUCTIONS

1 Preheat oven to 300° F.
2 In a saucepan over medium heat, combine coconut milk, honey, salt, seeds from scraped vanilla beans, and vanilla beans. Stir occasionally for 4 minutes, until steam rises, but do not boil. Discard vanilla beans.
3 In a blender, add yolks and blend on low for 10 seconds.
4 Slowly pour hot coconut milk mixture through the hole in the lid of the blender.
5 Blend constantly until all milk mixture is incorporated. Go slowly; adding the hot mixture too quickly will scramble the eggs.
6 Pour custard into four 6-ounce ramekins.

7 Place ramekins in a deep baking pan. Pour boiling water into pan until it's about halfway up the sides of the ramekins.
8 Bake 45 minutes. Remove from oven when the custard is slightly firm and a little jiggly in the center.
9 Cool for 1 hour on a wire rack, then cover with plastic wrap and cool overnight in fridge.
10 When ready to serve, sprinkle 1 teaspoon of maple sugar on top of each.
11 Using a kitchen torch (or the broiler of your oven), caramelize the tops.
12 Garnish with fresh berries and mint leaves as desired to serve.

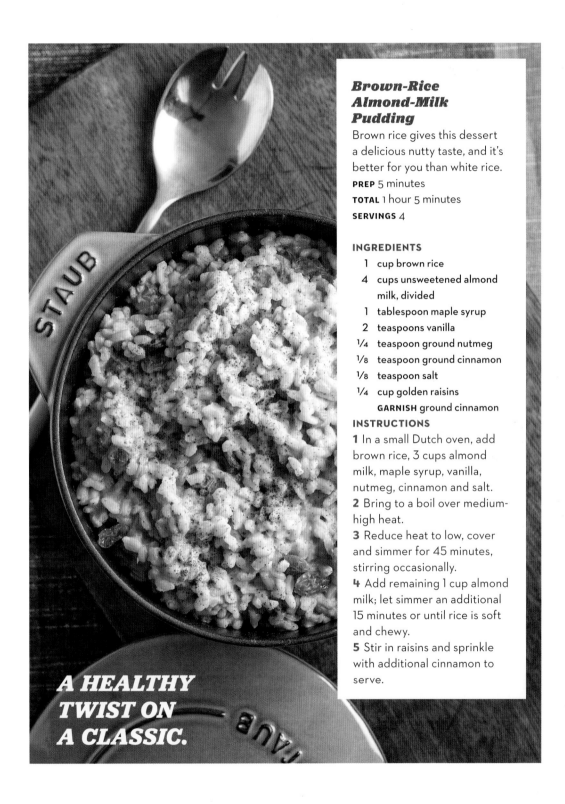

Brown-Rice Almond-Milk Pudding

Brown rice gives this dessert a delicious nutty taste, and it's better for you than white rice.

PREP 5 minutes

TOTAL 1 hour 5 minutes

SERVINGS 4

INGREDIENTS

- 1 cup brown rice
- 4 cups unsweetened almond milk, divided
- 1 tablespoon maple syrup
- 2 teaspoons vanilla
- ¼ teaspoon ground nutmeg
- ⅛ teaspoon ground cinnamon
- ⅛ teaspoon salt
- ¼ cup golden raisins
- **GARNISH** ground cinnamon

INSTRUCTIONS

1 In a small Dutch oven, add brown rice, 3 cups almond milk, maple syrup, vanilla, nutmeg, cinnamon and salt.

2 Bring to a boil over medium-high heat.

3 Reduce heat to low, cover and simmer for 45 minutes, stirring occasionally.

4 Add remaining 1 cup almond milk; let simmer an additional 15 minutes or until rice is soft and chewy.

5 Stir in raisins and sprinkle with additional cinnamon to serve.

A HEALTHY TWIST ON A CLASSIC.

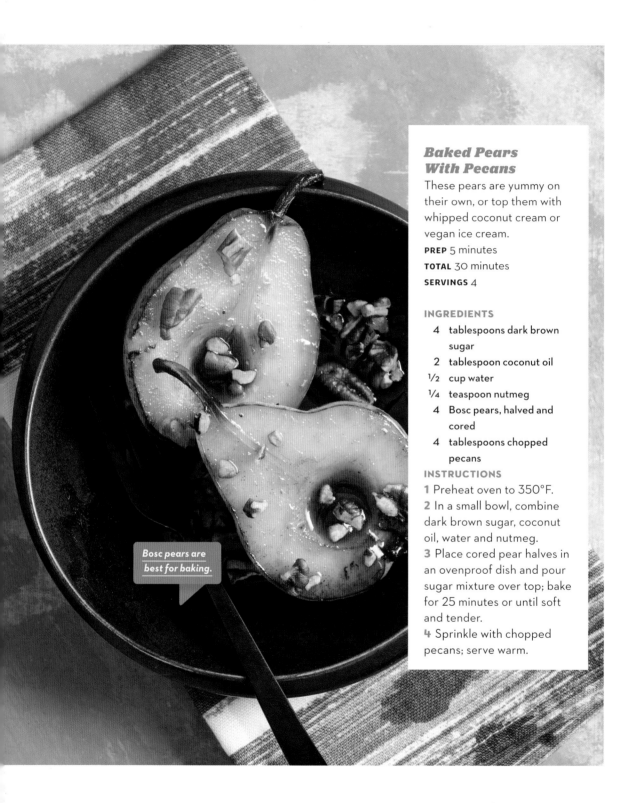

Bosc pears are best for baking.

Baked Pears With Pecans

These pears are yummy on their own, or top them with whipped coconut cream or vegan ice cream.

PREP 5 minutes
TOTAL 30 minutes
SERVINGS 4

INGREDIENTS

- 4 tablespoons dark brown sugar
- 2 tablespoon coconut oil
- ½ cup water
- ¼ teaspoon nutmeg
- 4 Bosc pears, halved and cored
- 4 tablespoons chopped pecans

INSTRUCTIONS

1 Preheat oven to 350°F.
2 In a small bowl, combine dark brown sugar, coconut oil, water and nutmeg.
3 Place cored pear halves in an ovenproof dish and pour sugar mixture over top; bake for 25 minutes or until soft and tender.
4 Sprinkle with chopped pecans; serve warm.

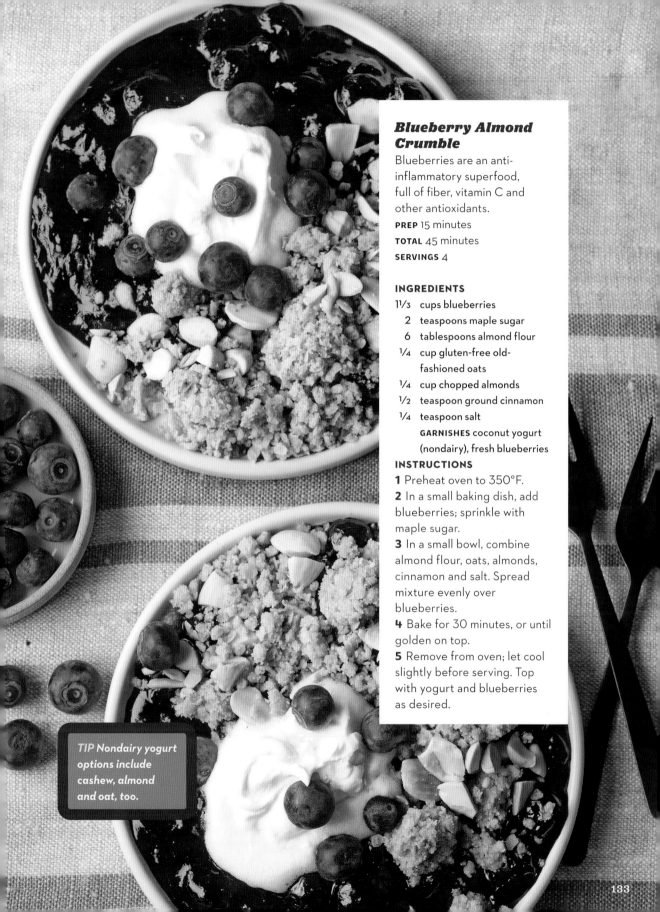

Blueberry Almond Crumble

Blueberries are an anti-inflammatory superfood, full of fiber, vitamin C and other antioxidants.

PREP 15 minutes
TOTAL 45 minutes
SERVINGS 4

INGREDIENTS

1⅓ cups blueberries
2 teaspoons maple sugar
6 tablespoons almond flour
¼ cup gluten-free old-fashioned oats
¼ cup chopped almonds
½ teaspoon ground cinnamon
¼ teaspoon salt
GARNISHES coconut yogurt (nondairy), fresh blueberries

INSTRUCTIONS

1 Preheat oven to 350°F.
2 In a small baking dish, add blueberries; sprinkle with maple sugar.
3 In a small bowl, combine almond flour, oats, almonds, cinnamon and salt. Spread mixture evenly over blueberries.
4 Bake for 30 minutes, or until golden on top.
5 Remove from oven; let cool slightly before serving. Top with yogurt and blueberries as desired.

TIP Nondairy yogurt options include cashew, almond and oat, too.

Apple Crisp With Coconut Cream

Whipped coconut cream keeps this crowd-pleasing dessert vegan—and oh-so-delicious!

PREP 10 minutes
TOTAL 55 minutes
+ 10 minutes inactive
SERVINGS 4

INGREDIENTS
Vegetable oil cooking spray
- ⅓ cup gluten-free almond flour
- ½ cup gluten-free old-fashioned oats
- ⅓ cup dark brown sugar
- ¾ teaspoon cinnamon, divided
- ⅛ teaspoon salt
- ¼ cup coconut oil
- 4 Granny Smith apples, peeled, cored and sliced
- ⅓ cup maple syrup
- ½ teaspoon ground cinnamon
- ⅛ teaspoon nutmeg
  Whipped coconut cream

INSTRUCTIONS
1 Preheat oven to 350°F. Grease an 8-inch-square baking pan with vegetable spray.
2 In a large bowl, combine flour, oats, brown sugar, ¼ teaspoon cinnamon, salt and coconut oil.
3 In another large bowl, toss apple slices, maple syrup, remaining cinnamon and nutmeg. Allow to sit for 10 minutes.
4 Place apple mixture in pan; sprinkle on oat mixture evenly.
5 Place pan on a baking sheet and bake for 45 minutes, or until topping is light golden brown and filling is bubbling.
6 Remove from oven; cool on wire rack for 10 minutes.
7 Serve warm with whipped coconut cream.

APPLES HAVE PRE- AND PROBIOTICS.

TIP *If you can't find coconut whipped cream in your store, don't fret—it's easy to make! Chill a 15-ounce can of full-fat coconut milk overnight. Scoop just the cream off the top (you can drink the remaining water). Use a hand mixer to beat until fluffy.*

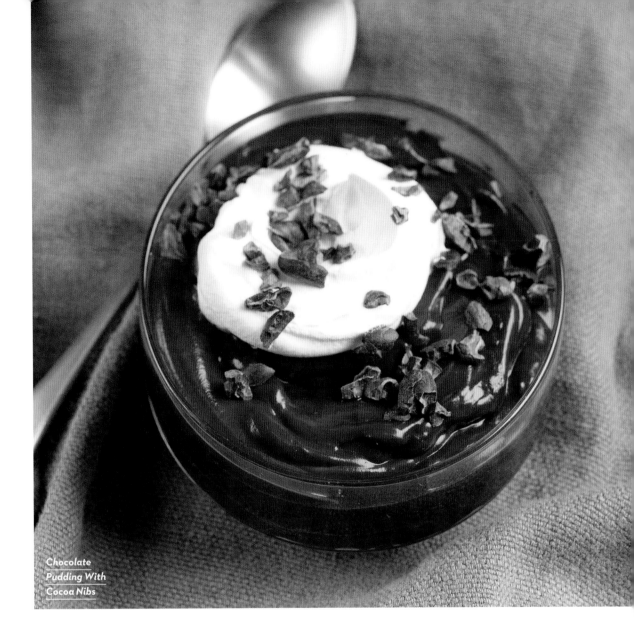

Chocolate Pudding With Cocoa Nibs

Chocolate Pudding With Cocoa Nibs

This is a super healthy dessert or snack option, thanks to chia seeds, protein powder and dark cocoa. Cocoa and cacao nibs are naturally low in sugar and maple syrup won't cause blood sugar to spike, so #guiltfree!

PREP 5 minutes

TOTAL 5 minutes + 1 hour inactive

SERVINGS 4

INGREDIENTS

2 cups unsweetened almond milk

6 tablespoons chia seeds

½ cup vegan chocolate protein powder

¼ cup dark cocoa powder

¼ cup maple syrup

GARNISHES whipped coconut cream, cocoa nibs

INSTRUCTIONS

1 In a blender, mix first 5 ingredients on high for 30 seconds.

2 Pour into 4 serving bowls; chill in refrigerator for about 1 hour. Garnish as desired and serve.

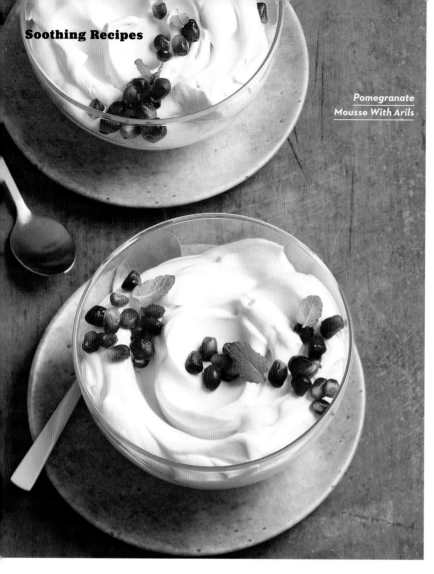

*Pomegranate
Mousse With Arils*

mixture. Stir with a whisk and let cool to room temperature.
4 Place thawed coconut cream in a large bowl; fold in gelatin mixture.
5 Pour into dessert bowls and chill until firm, about 4 hours.
6 Garnish with pomegranate arils and mint leaves.

Lemon Cheesecake Fat Bombs

These lemony treats are a tasty way to end a meal. Avoid if you are sensitive to dairy.
PREP 15 minutes
TOTAL 15 minutes,
+ 6 hours inactive
SERVINGS 18 bombs

INGREDIENTS
- ½ cup coconut oil
- ½ cup ghee
- ½ cup cultured cream cheese, softened
- 1 teaspoon lemon juice
- 1 teaspoon lemon zest
- 1 tablespoon honey
- ¼ teaspoon vanilla extract
- ⅛ teaspoon sea salt

INSTRUCTIONS
1 In a food processor, add coconut oil, ghee, cream cheese, lemon juice, zest, honey, vanilla and salt. Process until smooth.
2 Drop by rounded tablespoons on parchment paper.
3 Freeze for 6 hours; remove from freezer 5 minutes before serving.
4 Store in freezer for up to 3 months.

Pomegranate Mousse With Arils

Pomegranate seeds get their red hue from polyphenols, which are potent, inflammation-reducing antioxidants.
PREP 10 minutes
TOTAL 15 minutes
+ 4 hours inactive
SERVINGS 4

INGREDIENTS
- 1 cup pomegranate juice, divided
- 1 (¼-ounce) envelope gelatin
- 1 (9-ounce) container frozen coconut cream, thawed
  GARNISH pomegranate arils, mint leaves

INSTRUCTIONS
1 Pour ¼ cup pomegranate juice into a medium bowl; sprinkle gelatin over the top.
2 Let mixture sit for 5 minutes.
3 Meanwhile, heat remaining pomegranate juice in the microwave for 3 minutes. Pour hot juice over the gelatin

Toasted Coconut Panna Cotta

Coconut milk may help to reduce joint pain and curb inflammation.

PREP 25 minutes

TOTAL 25 minutes

+ 12 hours inactive

SERVINGS 4

INGREDIENTS

- 4 cups coconut milk, divided
- 1 (¼-ounce) envelope gelatin
- ⅓ cup honey
- 2 teaspoons vanilla
- **GARNISH** toasted coconut flakes

INSTRUCTIONS

1 In a small saucepan, pour 1 cup coconut milk; sprinkle evenly with gelatin. Let sit for 10 minutes to allow gelatin to soften.

2 Heat milk and gelatin over medium heat, stirring constantly, until gelatin is dissolved.

3 Stir remaining coconut milk and honey into the warm milk. Whisk until dissolved.

4 Remove from heat; stir in vanilla.

5 Let cool for 10 minutes and pour into 4 bowls.

6 Cover with plastic wrap and refrigerate overnight.

7 When ready to serve, garnish with toasted coconut flakes.

COCONUT MILK ALSO BALANCES THE GUT.

This dessert is also delicious with gluten-free shortbread!

Whipped Coconut Cream and Fruit Trifles

Assemble these ahead of time and keep in the fridge till ready to serve.

PREP 10 minutes
TOTAL 10 minutes
SERVINGS 4

INGREDIENTS

- 1 (9-ounce) container frozen coconut cream, thawed
- 1 cup raspberries
- 1 cup blueberries
- 1 cup strawberries, sliced
- 4 gluten-free oatmeal-chocolate chip cookies, crumbled

INSTRUCTIONS

1 In 4 individual glasses, layer coconut cream, berries and crumbled cookies (reserve some crumbles to sprinkle on top).

2 Repeat layers. Top with another dollop of cream.

3 Cover with plastic wrap and refrigerate several hours to set.

4 When ready to serve, garnish with remaining cookie crumbles.

Almond Milk Jelly Cups

Gelatin contains glutamic acid, which helps seal the digestive tract and reduce the risk of a leaky gut.

PREP 10 minutes

TOTAL 10 minutes
+ 4 hours inactive

SERVINGS 4

INGREDIENTS

2   cups almond milk, divided
4   teaspoons powdered gelatin
1   teaspoon honey
1   teaspoon vanilla extract

INSTRUCTIONS

1 In a small saucepan over low heat, add ½ cup almond milk and gelatin.
2 Whisk until gelatin is dissolved.
3 Remove from heat; add remaining almond milk, honey and vanilla and serve.

Vanilla Tapioca

Tapioca is a good option for those who may be prone to inflammation from foods containing gluten.

PREP 10 minutes

TOTAL 35 minutes

SERVINGS 4

INGREDIENTS

4   cups water
6   tablespoons quick tapioca
½   cup coconut crystals
2   teaspoons vanilla
¼   teaspoon sea salt
1⅓ cups coconut milk

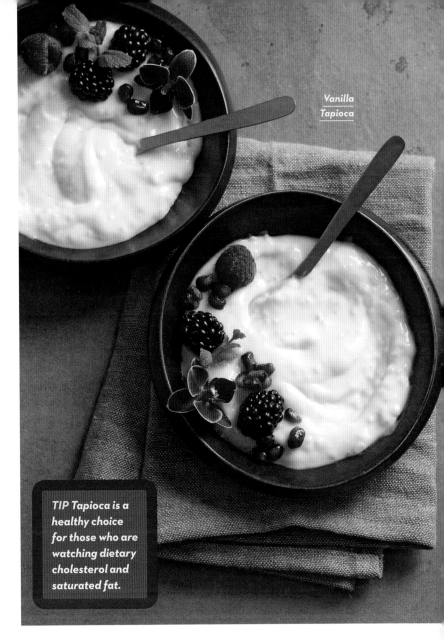

Vanilla Tapioca

TIP Tapioca is a healthy choice for those who are watching dietary cholesterol and saturated fat.

GARNISHES orchid blossoms, blackberries, raspberries, pomegranate arils

INSTRUCTIONS

1 In a medium saucepan, bring water to boil.
2 Whisk in tapioca. Let cook for 15 minutes, whisking occasionally.
3 In a medium bowl, whisk coconut crystals, vanilla, salt and milk.
4 Whisk milk mixture into tapioca and cook for 10 more minutes.
5 Pour mixture into 4 dessert bowls.
6 Garnish with orchid blossoms, berries and pomegranate arils.

SPECIAL THANKS TO CONTRIBUTING WRITERS

Brittany Risher Englert • Jacqueline Goodwin • Megan McMorris
Elizabeth Millard • Margaret Monroe • Kathryn Drury Wagner

CREDITS

CENTENNIAL BOOKS

An Imprint of
Centennial Media, LLC
1111 Brickell Avenue, 10th Floor
Miami, FL 33131, U.S.A.

CENTENNIAL BOOKS is a trademark of Centennial Media, LLC

ISBN 978-1-955703-11-6

Distributed by
Simon & Schuster, Inc.
1230 Avenue of the Americas
New York, NY 10020, U.S.A.

For information about custom editions, special sales and premium and corporate purchases, please contact Centennial Media at contact@centennialmedia.com.

Manufactured in China

© 2022 by Centennial Media, LLC

10 9 8 7 6 5 4 3 2 1

Publishers & Co-Founders Ben Harris, Sebastian Raatz
Editorial Director Annabel Vered
Creative Director Jessica Power
Executive Editor Janet Giovanelli
Design Director Martin Elfers
Features Editor Alyssa Shaffer
Deputy Editors Ron Kelly, Amy Miller Kravetz, Anne Marie O'Connor
Managing Editor Lisa Chambers
Senior Art Directors Lan Yin Bachelis, Pino Impastato
Art Directors Olga Jakim, Alberto Diaz, Jaclyn Loney, Natali Suasnavas, Joseph Ulatowski
Copy/Production Patty Carroll, Angela Taormina
Senior Photo Editor Jenny Veiga
Photo Editor Keri Pruett
Production Manager Paul Rodina
Production Assistants Tiana Schippa, Alyssa Swiderski
Editorial Assistants Michael Foster, Alexis Rotnicki
Sales & Marketing Jeremy Nurnberg